Infection, Ischemia, and Amputation

Guest Editor

MICHAEL S. PINZUR, MD

FOOT AND ANKLE CLINICS

www.foot.theclinics.com

Consulting Editor
MARK S. MYERSON, MD

September 2010 • Volume 15 • Number 3

SAUNDERS an imprint of ELSEVIER, Inc.

W.B. SAUNDERS COMPANY
A Division of Elsevier Inc.

1600 John F. Kennedy Blvd. ● Suite 1800 ● Philadelphia, PA 19103-2899

http://www.theclinics.com

FOOT AND ANKLE CLINICS Volume 15, Number 3
September 2010 ISSN 1083-7515, ISBN-13: 978-1-4377-2450-9

Editor: Debora Dellapena
Developmental Editor: Donald Mumford

Foot and Ankle Clinics (ISSN 1083-7515) is published quarterly by Elsevier, Inc., 360 Park Avenue South, New York, NY 10010-1710. Months of issue are March, June, September, and December. Periodicals postage paid at New York, NY, and additional mailing offices. Subscription price per year is $253.00 (US individuals), $340.00 (US institutions), $128.00 (US students), $283.00 (Canadian individuals), $402.00 (Canadian institutions), $175.00 (Canadian students), $364.00 (foreign individuals), $402.00 (foreign institutions), and $175.00 (foreign students). To receive student/resident rate, orders must be accompanied by name of affiliated institution, date of term, and the *signature* of program/residency coordinator on institution letterhead. Orders will be billed at individual rate until proof of status is received. Foreign air speed delivery is included in all *Clinics* subscription prices. All prices are subject to change without notice. **POSTMASTER:** Send address changes to *Foot and Ankle Clinics*, Elsevier Health Sciences Division, Subscription Customer Service, 3251 Riverport Lane, Maryland Heights, MO 63043. **Customer Service: 1-800-654-2452 (US and Canada). From outside of the United States and Canada, call 314-447-8871. Fax: 314-447-8029. E-mail: JournalsCustomerService-usa@ elsevier.com (for print support); JournalsOnlineSupport-usa@elsevier.com (for online support).**

Reprints. For copies of 100 or more, of articles in this publication, please contact the Commercial Reprints Department, Elsevier Inc., 360 Park Avenue South, New York, NY 10010-1710. Tel.: 212-633-3812; Fax: 212-462-1935; E-mail: reprints@elsevier.com.

Printed in the United States of America

Transferred to Digital Printing, 2011

Contributors

CONSULTING EDITOR

MARK S. MYERSON, MD
Director, The Institute for Foot and Ankle Reconstruction at Mercy, Mercy Medical Center, Baltimore, Maryland

GUEST EDITOR

MICHAEL S. PINZUR, MD
Professor of Orthopaedic Surgery & Rehabilitation, Loyola University Medical Center, Maywood, Illinois

AUTHORS

CHRISTOPHER E. ATTINGER, MD
Professor and Chief, Division of Wound Healing, Department of Plastic Surgery, Georgetown University Medical Center, Washington, DC

BERNADETTE AULIVOLA, MD, RVT
Assistant Professor, Departments of Surgery and Radiology, Stritch School of Medicine; Program Director, Fellowship in Vascular Surgery, Division of Vascular Surgery and Endovascular Therapy, Loyola University Medical Center, Maywood, Illinois

WAYNE S. BERBERIAN, MD
Associate Professor, Department of Orthopaedics, University of Medicine and Dentistry of New Jersey, New Jersey Medical School, Newark, New Jersey

ERIC A. BREITBART, MD
Resident, PGY-1, Department of Orthopaedics, University of Medicine and Dentistry of New Jersey, New Jersey Medical School, Newark, New Jersey

MARK W. CLEMENS, MD
Chief Resident, Department of Plastic Surgery, Georgetown University Medical Center, Washington, DC

ROBERT M. CRAIG, DO
Fellow, Division of Vascular Surgery and Endovascular Therapy, Loyola University Medical Center, Maywood, Illinois

DANIEL J. CUTTICA, DO
Fellow, Orthopedic Foot and Ankle Center, Westerville, Ohio

EMILY L. EXTEN, MD
Resident, Department of Orthopaedic Surgery, Medical College of Wisconsin, Milwaukee, Wisconsin

TOMIKO FUKUDA, MD
Fondren Orthopaedic Group LLC, Pearland, Texas

DENNIS J. JANISSE, CPed
Clinical Assistant Professor, Department of Rehabilitation and Physical Medicine, Medical College of Wisconsin; President and CEO, National Pedorthic Services Inc, Milwaukee, Wisconsin

ERICK J. JANISSE, CPed, CO
Vice President, National Pedorthic Services Inc, Saint Louis, Missouri

SHELDON S. LIN, MD
Associate Professor, Department of Orthopaedics, University of Medicine and Dentistry of New Jersey, New Jersey Medical School, Newark, New Jersey

FRANK A. LIPORACE, MD
Assistant Professor, Department of Orthopaedics, University of Medicine and Dentistry of New Jersey, New Jersey Medical School, Newark, New Jersey

JASON T. LONG, PhD
Assistant Professor, Department of Orthopaedic Surgery, Medical College of Wisconsin, Milwaukee; Orthopaedic and Rehabilitation Engineering Center (OREC), Marquette Uiversity, Medical College of Wisconsin, Wisconsin

RICHARD M. MARKS, MD, FACS
Director, Division of Foot and Ankle Surgery; Professor, Department of Orthopaedic Surgery, Medical College of Wisconsin, Milwaukee, Wisconsin

SIDDHANT K. MEHTA
Pre-doctoral Research Fellow, Department of Orthopaedics, University of Medicine and Dentistry of New Jersey, New Jersey Medical School, Newark, New Jersey

TERRENCE M. PHILBIN, DO
Assistant Clinical Professor, OSU Department of Orthopaedic Surgery, The Ohio State University College of Medicine and Public Health; Attending Physician, Orthopedic Foot and Ankle Center, Westerville, Ohio

MICHAEL S. PINZUR, MD
Professor of Orthopaedic Surgery and Rehabilitation, Loyola University Medical Center, Maywood, Illinois

AMY JO PTASZEK, MD
Clinical Instructor Orthopaedic Surgery, The University of Chicago, Chicago; Illinois Bone and Joint Institute, LTD, Glenview, Illinois

VERRABDHADRA REDDY, MD
Austin Othopaedics, Austin, Texas

RONALD A. SAGE, DPM
Professor and Chief, Section of Podiatry, Department of Orthopaedic Surgery and Rehabilitation, Loyola University Chicago, Stritch School of Medicine, Maywood; Staff Podiatrist, Edward Hines Jr Veterans Affairs Hospital, Hines, Illinois

Contents

Given the aging population, the number of patients at risk for peripheral arterial disease and critical limb ischemia will increase in the upcoming decade. Using a focused history and physical examination, along with a combination of noninvasive physiologic testing and noninvasive and invasive imaging modalities, one can accurately assess the location and physiologic effect of peripheral arterial disease. This assessment then allows the selection of the most appropriate treatment option for each patient. Treatment options may include exercise and risk-factor modification, amputation, and endovascular or surgical revascularization or a combination of both.

Impaired soft tissue regeneration and delayed osseous healing are known complications associated with diabetes mellitus with regard to orthopedic surgery, making the management and treatment of diabetic patients undergoing foot and ankle surgery more complex and difficult. At the moment several options are available to address the known issues that complicate the clinical outcomes in these high-risk patients. Using a multifaceted approach, with close attention to intraoperative and perioperative considerations including modification of surgical technique to supplement fixation, local application of orthobiologics, tight glycemic control, administration of supplementary oxygen, and biophysical stimulation via low-intensity pulsed ultrasound and electrical bone stimulation, the impediments associated with diabetic healing can potentially be overcome, to yield improved clinical results for diabetic patients after acute or elective foot and ankle surgery.

Successful foot and ankle reconstructions require a detailed knowledge of vascular anatomy. This knowledge becomes all the more important in diabetic patients because of healing complications and high incidence of peripheral vascular disease; it allows foot and ankle surgeons to design safe exposures and vascular surgeons to choose effective revascularization strategies. The angiosome concept separates the body into distinct threedimensional blocks of tissue fed by source arteries. This article focuses on the surgical implications of angiosomes of the foot and ankle and their arterial-arterial connections.

Diabetes mellitus is a common disease in the world today and its prevalence is increasing. Foot and ankle complications, including infection, are the most common reason for hospital admission in patients with diabetes mellitus in the United States and are commonly encountered by the foot and ankle surgeon. Thorough clinical examination with appropriate use of adjunctive laboratory and imaging studies can allow for early diagnosis and treatment, which can improve patient outcomes. Mild infections can often be treated on an outpatient basis with oral antibiotics and local debridement, whereas more severe infections require hospitalization, intravenous antibiotics, and surgical debridement to fully eradicate the infection. Despite proper treatment, amputation is still common in diabetics.

Infections in and around the calcaneus can be quite challenging for the patients and physicians involved. These infections arise because of multiple potential etiologies including chronic pressure, trauma, and postsurgical wound-healing complications. The impediments to healing can be equally as diverse depending on patients' comorbidities, such as smoking, diabetes, and open injury. In this article the authors review the anatomy of the calcaneus and surrounding soft tissue, patient risk factors, and various treatment options that can be used through a multidisciplinary approach. The common limiting factor for most of these patients is the delicate soft-tissue envelope, and occasionally, the lack thereof. The ultimate goal is an infection-free limb with durable soft-tissue coverage and maximal maintenance of function.

The Syme's ankle disarticulation is an end-bearing amputation level that provides stable walking, requires minimal physical therapy gait training, and rarely requires hospitalization on a rehabilitation unit. This article discusses patient selection, surgical technique, and rehabilitation of an underused rehabilitation amputation level.

Partial foot amputations are frequently performed to salvage significant portions of the lower extremity affected by limb-threatening infection.

Once healed, the residual foot is at high risk for reulceration. Careful long-term follow-up and appropriate interventions can lower this risk.

Amputations of the lower extremity may result from several etiologic factors. Most amputations performed in the United States result from a dysvascular limb. A majority of the population with vascular impairment comprises people with diabetes. These individuals frequently have comorbidities that may also affect the ultimate outcome of amputation. Loss of protective sensation, propensity toward infection, and visual and balance impairment all create additional issues with postamputation gait in the population with diabetes. Amputations about the foot and ankle affect gait and energy consumption. More gait disturbances tend to be seen as amputation level becomes more proximal; however, loss of the metatarsophalangeal joints has a profound effect, regardless of the proximal level of amputation. Soft tissue balance is key to maximizing gait, particularly prevention of equinus and equinovarus deformity from unopposed plantarflexors. Orthotic, prosthetic, and shoe modifications can help minimize gait abnormalities; however alterations of ground reaction force and center of pressure may still remain.

Amputations in patients with diabetes, while often preventable, are unfortunately a far too common outcome. The roles of the certified or licensed pedorthist, certified orthotist, and the certified prosthetist should not be undervalued in the prevention of diabetic foot complications (eg, amputations, revisions, and foot infections secondary to skin ulcerations) and in returning the patient a normal, active, and productive lifestyle in the event of an amputation. This article highlights the roles these specialists play in treating patients with partial foot amputation.

THE CLINICS ARE NOW AVAILABLE ONLINE!

Access your subscription at:
www.theclinics.com

Preface

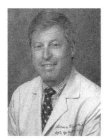

Michael S. Pinzur, MD
Guest Editor

This issue of *Foot and Ankle Clinics of North America* is dedicated to some of the most complex patients seen in an orthopedic practice: diabetics with lower extremity infection. The economic burden of diabetes in the United States may well be as high as $200 billion this year. More than 60,000 diabetics will undergo a lower extremity amputation this year. As many as a third of those will die within 2 years.

After World War II, Ernest Burgess popularized a new positive outcomes–oriented approach to the amputee. He stressed amputation surgery as constructive surgery, the first step in the rehabilitation of a patient with a nonsalvageable lower extremity, as opposed to failure mode surgery.

Modern peripheral vascular surgery and the appreciation of angiosomes have improved our ability to salvage limbs and preserve functional independence. Decision making based on outcomes expectations has improved our ability to optimize functional outcomes in this complex patient population.

The goal of this issue of *Foot and Ankle Clinics of North America* is to provide the reader with a background on the basic science of infection in this complex, highly morbid patient population and provide the modern approach to optimizing outcomes, whether or not that eventual end result is limb salvage or amputation. We have selected experts who understand that the goal of treatment is maximizing function as opposed to simply preserving tissue. Our goal is to modernize and change your viewpoint on this highly complex patient population.

Michael S. Pinzur, MD
Department of Orthopaedic Surgery and Rehabilitation
Loyola University Medical Center
2160 South First Avenue
Maywood, IL 60153, USA

E-mail address:
mpinzu1@lumc.edu

Foot Ankle Clin N Am 15 (2010) ix
doi:10.1016/j.fcl.2010.05.002
1083-7515/10/$ – see front matter © 2010 Elsevier Inc. All rights reserved.

foot.theclinics.com

Decision Making in the Dysvascular Lower Extremity

Bernadette Aulivola, MD, RVT[a,b,c,*], Robert M. Craig, DO[d]

KEYWORDS

• Dysvascular • Extremity • Ischemia

The presence of atherosclerotic peripheral arterial occlusive disease in patients with concomitant foot pathology often presents a challenge in clinical management strategy. Peripheral arterial disease (PAD) is a significant contributing factor in the occurrence and progression of foot pathology, especially in the diabetic patient population. Therefore, proper evaluation and management of the arterial flow to the foot in such instances is essential in efforts toward foot healing and foot salvage. This article aims to define the patient population at risk for PAD, describe the clinical presentation of such patients, and detail the appropriate evaluation and management of the dysvascular lower extremity in this setting.

SCOPE OF THE PROBLEM

The National Health and Nutritional Exam Survey evaluated in the United States a random sample of 2174 patients older than 40 years. Using ankle-brachial index (ABI) less than 0.90 as a definition of PAD, the prevalence of PAD in the study population was found to be 4.3%. When this percentage is extrapolated to the entire US population, it represents approximately 5 million people. The rate of PAD was found to be 14.5% in people older than 70 years.[1] Hirsch and colleagues[2] screened 6979 patients for PAD in the primary care setting. The patients were older than 70 years or between the ages of 50 and 69 years with significant risk factors for PAD, such as smoking or diabetes. The rate of peripheral vascular disease in this population

[a] Department of Surgery, Stritch School of Medicine, Loyola University Medical Center, 2160 South First Avenue, Maywood, IL 60153, USA
[b] Department of Radiology, Stritch School of Medicine, Loyola University Medical Center, 2160 South First Avenue, Maywood, IL 60153, USA
[c] Division of Vascular Surgery and Endovascular Therapy, Loyola University Medical Center, 2160 South First Avenue, Building 110, Room 3216, Maywood, IL 60153, USA
[d] Division of Vascular Surgery and Endovascular Therapy, Loyola University Medical Center, 2160 South First Avenue, Building 110, Maywood, IL 60153, USA
* Corresponding author. Division of Vascular Surgery and Endovascular Therapy, Loyola University Medical Center, 2160 South First Avenue, Building 110, Room 3216, Maywood, IL 60153.
E-mail address: baulivola@lumc.edu

Foot Ankle Clin N Am 15 (2010) 391–409
doi:10.1016/j.fcl.2010.03.004
1083-7515/10/$ – see front matter. Published by Elsevier Inc.

foot.theclinics.com

was found to be 29%. These studies demonstrate the high prevalence of PAD, especially in the aging population.

A wide range of symptoms can be seen in patients with PAD, depending on the severity of occlusive disease and the activity level of the patient. Patients who are relatively inactive may have asymptomatic PAD. Symptoms such as lower extremity fatigue, cramping, or pain with walking, also known as intermittent claudication, are often categorized as lifestyle limiting or nonlifestyle limiting for the purposes of clinical management decision making. More severe signs or symptoms of PAD are often referred to as critical limb ischemia (CLI), which includes ischemic foot pain at rest or foot ulceration or gangrene.

Several large population studies have evaluated the incidence of mild PAD symptoms such as intermittent claudication. At age 40 years, the prevalence rate is approximately 3%, but this rises to 6% by age 60 years. It has also been noted that between 10% and 50% of patients with intermittent claudication symptoms never seek medical treatment for their condition.[3]

The incidence of CLI has been evaluated using prospective population studies and via indirect evidence gleaned from amputation rates and studies looking at disease progression in CLI. At present, the rate of CLI in developed countries is 500 to 1000 cases per million population per year.[3] Acute limb ischemia (ALI) is a sudden decrease in limb perfusion, usually threatening limb viability. There are little data on the incidence of ALI, but several national vascular registries suggest that the incidence is about 140 cases per million population per year.[3]

The entry of the baby boomer population into the age group at risk for PAD, combined with increasing rates of obesity and diabetes mellitus, seems to indicate that the incidence of PAD will continue to increase in the upcoming years. The continued use of cigarettes and other tobacco products only compounds the problem of PAD.

PATHOGENESIS

A basic understanding of the pathogenesis of atherosclerotic arterial occlusive disease is crucial in understanding the principles of evaluation and management of this condition. Risk factors for development of atherosclerotic disease include hypertension, family history of atherosclerosis, hyperhomocysteinemia, hyperlipidemia, smoking, and diabetes mellitus. The presence of one or more of these risk factors influences the anatomic location of disease and atherosclerotic plaque characteristics.[4] Overall, the superficial femoral artery is the most commonly affected lower extremity artery. Smoking and hyperlipidemia predispose to atherosclerotic disease in the aortoiliac and superficial femoral arteries.

Diabetic patients, especially nonsmokers, typically have atherosclerotic disease confined to the tibial arteries below the knee. In this patient group, the foot vessels are often spared of disease. Diabetic patients have a 4-fold higher prevalence of atherosclerosis and a 15-fold higher incidence of lower extremity amputation than the nondiabetic population.[5] Tibial artery plaque localization in patients with diabetes is thought to be related to the inability of the smooth muscle cells of these arteries to relax in response to pharmacologic and physiologic stimuli. The smooth muscle cells in these arteries proliferate in response to elevated levels of insulin and glucose.[6]

CLINICAL PRESENTATION OF THE DYSVASCULAR EXTREMITY

The dysvascular lower extremity can be divided into 2 broad categories based on the timing and presentation of the ischemia: acute and chronic. Chronic limb ischemia can further be divided into 3 categories that represent a spectrum of arterial disease: asymptomatic, intermittent claudication, or CLI.

Acute Limb Ischemia

ALI is defined as any sudden decrease in limb perfusion causing a potential threat to limb viability.[3] Typically, this sudden decrease in perfusion is caused by a worsening of existing PAD, thrombosis of a diseased arterial segment, or embolism to the peripheral vasculature, usually from a cardiac source, in a previously asymptomatic patient. The timeline of patient presentation from the onset of symptoms can vary depending on the cause of the acute occlusion. Patients suffering from an embolism to a peripheral arterial domain generally appear within hours of the inciting event. Patients with thrombosis of a previously diseased atherosclerotic arterial segment may have less severe symptoms and may not seek care for several days or weeks because their occlusion is better tolerated given the presence of more developed arterial collaterals associated with their chronic arterial occlusive disease.

On evaluation, the acutely ischemic limb is placed into one of 3 general categories: viable, immediately threatened, or nonviable. Examination may reveal some or all of the classic 6 p's of ALI: pain, pallor, pulselessness, paresthesias, poikilothermia, and paralysis. Muscle paralysis and sensory deficit to the leg are late findings and indicate severe ischemia with impending muscle and nerve function loss. The extremity may initially appear white but progresses to a mottled appearance. Progression to a fixed bluish discoloration often indicates a nonviable extremity. Initial treatment of ALI is systemic anticoagulation with heparin. This treatment is done to prevent the propagation of thrombus in the affected extremity. The workup of ALI may include imaging with duplex ultrasound, digital subtraction angiography (DSA), computed tomography angiography (CTA), or magnetic resonance angiography (MRA). As time is of essence, in many cases of ALI, arteriography is often performed in the operating room along with limb revascularization. Treatment options for ALI include catheter-directed thrombolytic therapy, percutaneous aspiration thrombectomy, percutaneous mechanical thrombectomy, surgical thrombectomy, and surgical bypass. Multiple studies have shown no difference in outcomes between catheter-directed thrombolytic therapy and conventional surgery in the patient population with ALI.[7,8] Patients who present with ALI have a 30-day major amputation rate of 10% to 30%.[3]

Chronic Limb Ischemia

Atherosclerosis is the most common cause of chronic limb ischemia. However, other rare conditions including popliteal artery entrapment syndrome, mucinous cystic degeneration, abdominal aortic coarctation, Buerger disease, fibrodysplastic disease, persistent sciatic artery, iliac artery syndrome of the cyclist, and primary arterial tumors warrant mention and should be considered as possible causes of ischemia in patients without typical risk factors for atherosclerotic disease.

Chronic atherosclerotic PAD manifests as a continuum of signs and symptoms that can be divided into 3 categories, in order of increasing severity: asymptomatic, intermittent claudication, and CLI, which includes ischemic rest pain and tissue loss. These categories represent the normal evolution of symptoms in the population with PAD. This sequence of progression may differ in the diabetic population as a result of the effects of diabetic neuropathy. Not all patients with PAD go through a sequential progression of symptoms, and often the first sign of PAD is the nonhealing foot ulceration or gangrenous lesion.

Intermittent claudication

Intermittent claudication is an important early sign of PAD and should always be elicited in a patient's medical history. Claudication is defined as ischemic muscle pain that occurs as a result of inadequate blood flow during periods of activity. This poor tissue perfusion is the result of proximal arterial occlusive disease, resulting in insufficient blood flow to meet the metabolic needs of the large muscle groups of the lower extremities during exercise. Intermittent claudication of the thighs and buttocks typically occurs as the result of occlusive disease of the aortoiliac system. Intermittent claudication of the lower leg is a more common presenting symptom of PAD and is characterized by fatigue or cramping pain in the calves that occur with activity, such as walking. The symptoms are not present at rest but develop progressively as the patient walks and usually cause the patient to stop walking after a predictable distance or time. After stopping to rest, the patient typically experiences relief of the pain or discomfort within several minutes and can then walk a similar distance before being forced to stop again because of recurrence of symptoms. In early disease, the symptoms may only manifest when the patient is walking up a grade or at a fast pace and may be absent when walking on level ground at a slow speed. Intermittent claudication is typically quantified by the distance that the patient can walk before being forced to stop, usually expressed in either city blocks or, in more severe cases, feet. Documentation of this distance is useful in following the progression of the disease and can help identify patients with worsening occlusive disease before the appearance of more severe symptoms, such as ischemic rest pain or tissue loss.

Most patients with PAD are asymptomatic or have only mild claudication symptoms. Fortunately, claudication is often associated with a favorable natural history. The prevalence of intermittent claudication is approximately 3% in patients aged 40 years and increases to 6% in those aged 60 years.[9] Only 25% of patients with claudication symptoms develop clinical progression over time, and only 20% require extremity revascularization at 10 years. The lower extremity amputation rate in patients with claudication is low at 1% to 3% at 5 years.[9] However, in smokers and patients with diabetes, the natural history of claudication can be less favorable.

Critical limb ischemia

CLI was defined by the TransAtlantic Intersociety Consensus (TASC) Conference as persistent ischemic rest pain of the foot for at least 2 weeks, or ulceration or gangrene of the foot or toes, and ankle systolic pressure of less than 50 mm Hg or toe systolic pressure of less than 30 mm Hg.[10] Amputation is the primary treatment for up to 25% of patients with CLI.[9]

Ischemic rest pain is characterized as pain involving the forefoot or the region over the metatarsal heads and toes. Unlike intermittent claudication, ischemic rest pain is constant and, as its name implies, is not related to activity but occurs at rest. This symptom implies that the arterial supply is inadequate to meet the metabolic needs of the extremity tissue at rest, and in general, does not occur unless at least 2 separate regions of significant arterial stenosis or occlusion are present within the extremity. Patients often complain of exacerbation of ischemic rest pain symptoms at night, when the foot is elevated in bed and gravity-assisted blood flow augmentation is not in effect. They typically dangle the affected leg over the side of the bed at night to gain symptomatic relief. Diabetic patients may not develop rest pain, or the symptoms may easily be confused with those of peripheral neuropathy, subsequently delaying the diagnosis of severe foot ischemia in this subgroup of patients.

Tissue loss is the most severe presentation of PAD and may present in 2 distinct forms: foot ulceration and tissue necrosis, also known as gangrene. Foot ulceration usually involves the bony prominences of the lower extremities, such as the heads of the first or fifth metatarsal and the posterior aspect of the heel. In the presence of decreased arterial perfusion pressure in the extremity, even mild pressure at these locations can cause tissue necrosis and ulceration. Patients presenting with foot ulceration are often diabetic. Multiple factors, such as the presence of foot deformity and peripheral neuropathy, contribute to the increased incidence of foot ulceration in this subgroup of patients. All patients presenting with foot ulceration or gangrene should undergo prompt evaluation for PAD because these symptoms constitute what is known as CLI, and the risk for resultant limb loss is significant if arterial disease is not addressed. The gangrenous extremity is a hallmark of severe arterial occlusive disease. The diagnosis of gangrene is relatively straightforward on physical examination. On inspection, the involved extremity is black and shriveled, is insensate, and has no motor function. Without the presence of coexisting infection, gangrene is of little systemic consequence; however, this is not true when gangrenous tissue becomes secondarily infected, resulting in wet gangrene. This separate clinical entity is characterized by the gangrenous extremity associated with signs and symptoms of invasive infection, including fever, chills, leukocytosis, erythema, cellulitis, purulent drainage, abscess, and osteomyelitis. Unlike its uninfected counterpart, wet gangrene constitutes a surgical emergency.

EVALUATION FOR PAD

The evaluation of the patient with the dysvascular lower extremity begins with a comprehensive history and physical examination. Evaluation is then further supported by various noninvasive and invasive tests. These diagnostic modalities, which include the ABI, pulse volume recordings (PVRs), segmental arterial pressures, toe pressures, transcutaneous oxygen pressure ($tcPo_2$) measurements, CTA, MRA, and DSA, provide various physiologic and anatomic data to the clinician. Although DSA remains the gold standard in the assessment of peripheral arterial occlusive disease, the noninvasive modalities are preferred for the initial screening and workup of patients with PAD.

The diagnosis of vascular insufficiency in the lower extremity can usually be made on the basis of the patient's history and physical examination. Key points in the patient's history include walking distance and any symptoms of claudication or rest pain. Leriche syndrome, characterized by a history of erectile dysfunction, bilateral hip and buttock claudication, leg muscle atrophy, and absence of femoral pulses, indicates aortoiliac occlusive disease. A full cardiovascular history is essential in this group of patients, as most will eventually succumb to either cerebrovascular or cardiovascular events. Risk factors for PAD, such as hypertension, diabetes, hyperlipidemia, and smoking, should be documented.

Physical Examination

Physical examination should start with recording of the patient's pulse and the blood pressure in both arms. The examination continues with auscultation of the neck and abdomen for audible bruits. Palpation of the abdomen in search of an abdominal aortic aneurysm should also be performed. Peripheral pulse examination is essential to the evaluation of the dysvascular extremity. In the lower extremity, the femoral pulses are usually easily palpated, if present, just below the inguinal ligament and about 2 fingerbreadths lateral to the pubic tubercle. More difficult to palpate are the pulses in the popliteal artery, which is best done with the examiner's fingertips gently hooked into the popliteal space from either side, with the knee slightly bent and the patient completely relaxing the leg. The dorsalis pedis artery, a terminal branch of the anterior tibial artery, is palpated on the dorsum of the foot, just lateral to the tendon of the extensor hallucis longus. The posterior tibial artery is found just posterior to the medial malleolus. Palpable pulses are generally documented as normal, diminished, or absent or by a number grading system (0, absent; 1+, diminished; 2+, normal; 3+, prominent). The feet and legs should be inspected for any signs of ulceration or gangrene. Dependent rubor, caused by gravity-induced dilatation of the cutaneous circulation, and elevation pallor after 1 to 2 minutes of elevation of the foot to 45° are important clinical signs of the dysvascular lower extremity. Provoking these changes on examination is known as Buerger test. The absence of palpable pulses in the dorsalis pedis and posterior tibial arteries indicates advanced occlusive disease and is a good predictor of the ultimate need for angiography, especially in the setting of tissue loss, poor wound healing, or gangrene. Pulse palpation alone has been demonstrated to be unreliable in the accurate diagnosis of PAD, especially in the busy clinic setting. One study documented a 19% underdiagnosis of PAD, when a pulse was reported as palpable in the setting of a reduced ABI, and a 34% overdiagnosis of PAD, when a pulse was reported as nonpalpable when it should have been based on ABI.[11]

Noninvasive Studies

When the distal pulses are nonpalpable on physical examination, insonation with a continuous-wave hand-held Doppler probe should be performed. The signals produced are typically characterized as triphasic, biphasic, or monophasic. Triphasic signals indicate normal lower extremity arteries, whereas biphasic signals indicate moderate disease and monophasic signals indicate severe arterial occlusion. In the most severe cases of arterial occlusive disease, the absence of audible arterial signals may be noted.

Noninvasive evaluation can often yield a significant amount of information regarding the location and severity of arterial occlusive disease. The ABI compares the systolic pressure of the upper extremity to that of the lower extremity. A thorough evaluation of any patient with suspected peripheral arterial disease should always include measurement of the ABI. The ABI is obtained using a handheld continuous-wave Doppler probe and a blood pressure cuff. After the patient has rested for several minutes in the supine position, the systolic pressure of the brachial artery in both arms is measured using the Doppler probe. Next, the systolic pressure in the dorsalis pedis and anterior tibial arteries is measured with the blood pressure cuff placed just above the ankle. To calculate the index, the higher of the 2 pressures in each foot (dorsalis pedis or posterior tibial) is divided by the higher of the pressures in the 2 arms (left or right). An ABI of less than 1.0 indicates impaired blood flow to that lower extremity. Patients with claudication typically have an ABI between 0.4 and 0.9. An ABI of less than 0.4 is usually found in patients presenting with ischemic rest pain and tissue loss. The ABI is of limited usefulness in the diabetic population because of the presence of arterial wall medial calcification in the arteries of the leg. This calcification causes the affected arteries to be less compressible than the brachial artery at the same pressure. As a result, the ABI measurement is falsely elevated, often yielding an ABI value of greater than 1.0, and is therefore unreliable in predicting the extent of PAD. In some cases, the arterial calcification can be so severe that the arteries cannot be occluded with a blood pressure cuff at all. Therefore, ABI measurements have little clinical application in the diabetic patient.

Segmental pressure measurement, which is the technique of measuring arterial pressures from the high thigh down to the foot, is an excellent method for assessing the location of occlusive arterial lesions that are severe enough to reduce the arterial pressure (**Fig. 1**). The test is performed by placing a series of pressure cuffs at various levels along the affected extremity. Systolic pressure measurements are then taken at each level and correspond to the tissue perfusion at that level. A decrease in pressure between adjacent levels indicates the presence of an occlusive lesion within the intervening arterial segment. Similarly, comparing the pressures recorded in the same segment in both legs may indicate that an arterial stenosis is present in the leg with the lower pressure. As with ABIs, the segmental pressure measurements are also affected by the arterial wall calcification found in patients with diabetes, making this test unreliable in this patient population.

PVRs assess the flow characteristics within the arterial system (**Fig. 2**). A series of air plethysmography cuffs are placed along the extremity. These cuffs detect the small change in volume of the leg between systole and diastole and record these findings as a waveform. A progression from a triphasic to a monophasic or dampened waveform indicates occlusive disease. One advantage of PVR is that it is not affected by arterial wall calcification, as is segmental pressure measurement. Standardized amplitude measurements using this technique are problematic because they can be affected by factors such as cardiac output, vasomotor tone, and the gain settings of the recording equipment. Therefore, this test is generally interpreted as a qualitative examination of the waveform, making it difficult to use it as an absolute determinant of disease severity.

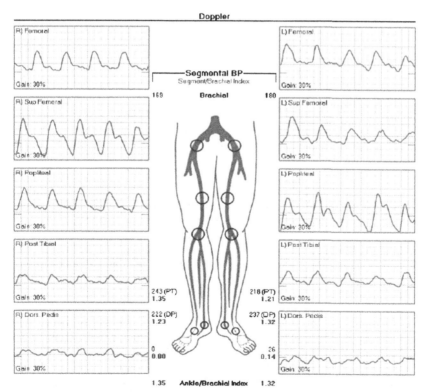

Fig. 1. Segmental blood pressure (BP) recording. This recording was done in a diabetic patient with noncompressible vessels. Note that the ABIs are greater than 1 despite disease in the dorsalis pedis (DP) and posterior tibial (PT) arteries.

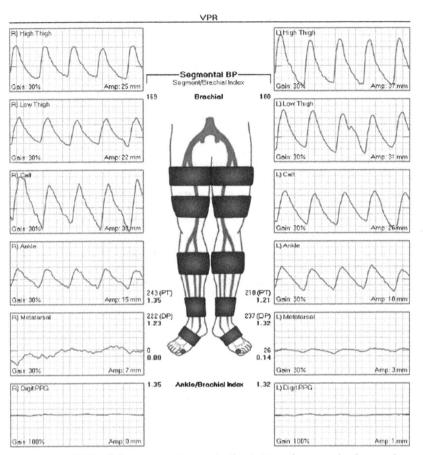

Fig. 2. Segmental PVR of the same patient as in **Fig. 1.** Note the severely abnormal waveforms at the metatarsal and digital levels. DP, dorsalis pedis; PPG, photoplethysmography; PT, posterior tibial.

TcPo$_2$ measurements have also been used to evaluate the amount of tissue perfusion in patients with peripheral arterial disease. This method indirectly measures the oxygen tension in the underlying tissue and has been used to predict the healing potential of the diseased extremity in cases of an existing wound or a potential wound, such as one created by performing a surgical procedure. The test is performed by placing a probe over the metatarsal region of the affected foot. After equilibrating the probe to a specific temperature, the oxygen tension of the skin is determined. Enthusiasm for this test has been tempered by the large degree of variability noted in the measurements obtained. Many factors, including the site of measurement, the ambient temperature, local infection, and extremity edema, are thought to affect the tcPo$_2$ reading. However, on review of multiple factors, no one factor was noted to account for the variability in measurement.[12] Another review noted that the tcPo$_2$ measurements were lower in diabetic patients than in nondiabetic patients when comparing groups with similar arterial disease severity.[13] Although there exists literature supporting the use of tcPo$_2$ measurements in the foot of patients with diabetes,[14] results are difficult to interpret. This has led to a gray zone of measurements without significant predictive value. The continued evaluation of this modality may lead to a better understanding of its role in the evaluation of the ischemic extremity. As mentioned earlier, noncompressible vessels resulting from arterial wall calcification, found especially in the diabetic patient population, can render pressure readings in the lower extremities nondiagnostic. However, it has been found that the vessels of the foot are largely spared the atherosclerotic changes noted in the more proximal arterial segments. Therefore, the measurement of toe pressures has become a useful adjunct in evaluating patients with noncompressible leg arteries. Toe pressures are measured with small (2–3 cm) cuffs placed on the great toe. The toe-brachial index (TBI) is normally less than the ABI, with a normal TBI being 0.65 or higher. Multiple studies suggest that an absolute toe pressure greater than 30 to 40 mm Hg is required to heal a wound in the foot. One study of the prognostic value of toe pressures documented that foot ulceration was not healed in any patient in the study group primarily if the toe pressure was less than 40 mm Hg.[15] In this study, primary foot healing was achieved in 85% of patients with toe pressure greater than 45 mm Hg and only in 36% with toe pressure less than 45 mm Hg. It has been demonstrated elsewhere that toe pressure is an accurate hemodynamic indicator of peripheral arterial occlusive disease in the diabetic patient population.[16] Although this methodology can be a useful adjunct in the evaluation of vascular disease and potential wound healing in diabetic patients, its use is at times problematic in these patients because of the presence of ulceration, gangrene, or previous toe amputation.

Duplex ultrasound examination of the arteries is a noninvasive, reproducible study that combines gray-scale B-mode imaging and pulsed wave color Doppler (**Fig. 3**). Using the gray-scale imaging, the arteries and any significant plaques within the lumen can be visualized. Doppler interrogation of the visualized artery can then be performed, giving information about flow through the artery. Spectral analysis of the Doppler waveform can detect stenosis and turbulent flow within an arterial segment. Stenosis within the artery causes increased blood flow velocity, which can be measured as the peak systolic velocity. This value is compared with the velocity in the artery proximal to the area of stenosis. This ratio, the V2/V1 ratio, can then be used to gauge the degree of stenosis in the artery. A V2/V1 ratio of 2.0 indicates a luminal diameter narrowing of 50%, and a ratio of 4.0 indicates a 75% luminal diameter narrowing. The accuracy of the examination is highly operator dependent, relying on the expertise of the ultrasonographer to maintain the proper angle of insonation and to accurately orient the sampling cursor in the direction of arterial flow.

Invasive Testing

DSA has long been considered the gold standard in the evaluation of patients with PAD (**Fig. 4**). If a patient qualifies for invasive therapeutic intervention, angiography is performed in most cases, either preoperatively for open surgical revascularization or before and during an endovascular catheter-based treatment.[3] Intra-arterial DSA is a simple and effective methodology.[17] The images of conventional angiography have been greatly enhanced with the introduction of DSA. By digitally subtracting the bone and soft tissue components of the image, better visualization of the intra-arterial dye column is obtained. The radiographer can follow the contrast bolus over a greater period and select the optimal images, which results in improved visualization of the distal vasculature. DSA provides high-quality images of the distal vascular system, which are indispensable for operative planning before any bypass procedure. Because the procedure is invasive, there is potential morbidity associated with it. Known complications include puncture-site hematoma, pseudoaneurysm, or arteriovenous fistula as well as distal embolization and access artery thrombosis. Another area of concern when

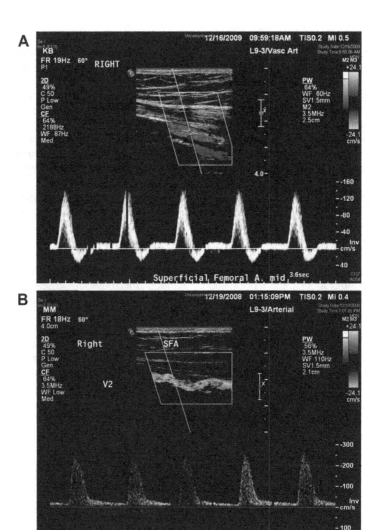

Fig. 3. Duplex ultrasound images of the superficial femoral artery (SFA). (*A*) Normal artery with triphasic spectral waveform. (*B*) Stenotic artery with spectral broadening of the waveform secondary to turbulent flow and high velocities.

performing angiography is the risk of nephrotoxicity from contrast agents, especially in patients with preexisting renal insufficiency. Careful consideration should be given to the type and amount of contrast medium used. Different options include carbon dioxide gas and ionic and nonionic contrast agents. Data in the literature show mixed conclusions regarding the incidence of nephrotoxicity related to various contrast agents. Although initial studies showed reduced nephrotoxicity associated with iso-osmolar nonionic contrast,[18] recent prospective randomized evidence shows that there is no difference in the incidence of contrast-induced nephropathy at 48 to 72 hours between groups of patients given either low-osmolar or iso-osmolar contrast media.[19] Of key importance is the recognition that many patients with PAD and diabetes also have renal insufficiency. An important factor in the prevention of renal failure in these patients is the use of intravenous hydration before and after contrast angiography.[20] In concert with

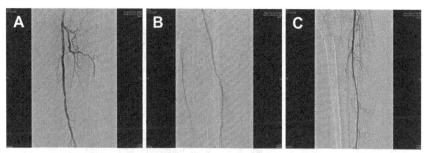

Fig. 4. Intra-arterial DSA in a patient with PAD. (*A*) Proximal superficial femoral artery with several areas of stenosis and profunda femoris artery. (*B*) Popliteal artery. (*C*) Below-knee runoff showing disease of the anterior and posterior tibial arteries and flow in the peroneal artery.

periprocedural hydration, the oral administration of the antioxidant *N*-acetylcysteine has been shown to prevent reduction in renal function caused by contrast agents in patients with underlying renal insufficiency.[21] If renal failure does occur after contrast angiography, it is almost always reversible with supportive care.[22] Iodinated contrast material can initiate a severe lactic acidosis in patients taking the oral medication metformin for glycemic control, which is especially true in those patients with decreased baseline renal function. Patients taking metformin should hold this medication for at least 48 hours before the administration of iodinated contrast. In general, patients on systemic anticoagulation with warfarin should stop this medication several days before angiography to allow their international normalized ratio to return to normal. Depending on the individual situation and the reason for anticoagulation, patients can be treated with heparin infusion or subcutaneous injections of low-molecular-weight heparin as a bridge off and on warfarin, if indicated. Antiplatelet agents such as aspirin and clopidogrel can generally be safely continued up until the time of angiography; however, the risks and benefits of their use must be individualized to each patient's clinical situation.

Other Imaging Options

CTA has improved in quality in recent years with the introduction of multislice helical scanners (**Fig. 5**). A volume of tissue is scanned, and the imaging information obtained is stored as voxels. Using computer imaging software, these voxels can then be reconstructed into 2-dimensional images that appear like regular DSA images and into 3-dimensional reconstructions that can be rotated on any axis. Some reviews have reported an accuracy of 95% to 99% when compared with DSA.[23,24] Despite this reported accuracy, there are several drawbacks to the use of CTA. Exposure to radiation and iodinated contrast material occurs during the examination. Interpretation of CTA is inaccurate in instances of overlapping leg veins. Existing intravascular stents can produce artifacts on CTA. Calcification can lead to artifact, making it difficult to evaluate calcified segments of vessel. CTA is also limited by the amount of contrast required to image the vasculature from the distal aorta to the foot. The combination of inaccuracy with calcification and the inability to visualize the pedal vessels makes CTA a less-than-optimal imaging modality for the evaluation of vascular disease in the diabetic population. One main advantage of DSA over CTA is the ability to perform diagnostic and therapeutic intervention in the same setting.

MRA is becoming an increasingly popular modality for the evaluation of the vasculature of the lower extremity. The technique has been found to be highly accurate in

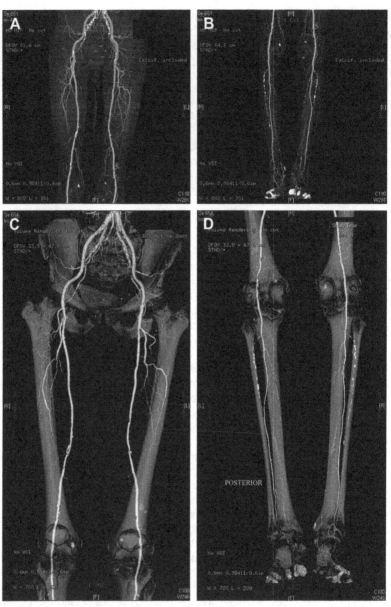

Fig. 5. CTA of the same patient as in **Fig. 4**. (*A*) Several areas of stenosis are seen in the superficial femoral artery. (*B*) Significant calcification and stenosis of the anterior and posterior tibial arteries. The peroneal artery is seen as the main runoff to the foot. (*C, D*) Three-dimensional volume rendering.

the assessment of lower extremity arterial disease, particularly with three-dimensional contrast-enhanced images.[25] MRA is an attractive option for imaging the arterial vasculature in the setting of contraindications for contrast dye. Evaluation of the utility of MRA has demonstrated more than 70% agreement with standard DSA findings in patients with lower extremity arterial occlusive disease when studied prospectively.[26]

TREATMENT OF THE DYSVASCULAR EXTREMITY

The presence of peripheral arterial occlusive disease predicts the presence of coronary occlusive disease in nearly all patients. One must take into consideration that mortality rates for patients with limb ischemia is elevated because of the concomitant presence of coronary and cerebrovascular disease. Mortality rates of up to 70% at 5 years have been observed in the patient population with CLI, often secondary to cardiac comorbidities. Therefore, modification of risk factors is of utmost importance in the treatment of the patient with dysvascular lower extremity, which includes efforts at smoking cessation, anticoagulation for treatment of hypercoagulable disorders, tight control of glucose levels in diabetic patients, and control of hypertension and hyperlipidemia. Antiplatelet agents are generally indicated in this patient group to reduce the risks of cardiac and cerebrovascular events. Clopidogrel has been demonstrated to be associated with a reduction in incidence of stroke, myocardial infarction, and death related to vascular causes, even when compared with the effects of aspirin alone.[27] These effects are particularly pronounced in the population with PAD. Patients with CLI and all patients with diabetes should be educated on daily foot examination and preventative foot care. The care of these patients is often dependent upon a multidisciplinary treatment approach to control the patient's pain, manage concomitant cardiovascular risk factors, and avoid limb loss. A basic algorithm exists for the evaluation and treatment of patients with the dysvascular lower extremity (**Fig. 6**).

Intermittent Claudication

In patients with intermittent claudication, initial management should be aimed at lifestyle modification and the implementation of a routine walking exercise program. These patients should be advised to undertake an exercise regimen consisting of walking up to 60 minutes per day for 3 times per week or more. Patients are typically instructed to walk until their symptoms cause them to stop, take a rest as needed, and continue walking. Supervised walking regimens have been demonstrated in many randomized trials to improve absolute claudication distance. When compared with control groups, patients who underwent exercise rehabilitation programs improved their absolute claudication distance by up to 200 meters more.[28] Smokers should be encouraged to stop smoking, and referral to a smoking cessation program may be of some benefit. Medical management of claudication has had mixed results, and currently only 2 medications are approved by the US Food and Drug Administration for this purpose. These medications include cilostazol and pentoxifylline. When walking regimens, medical management, and smoking cessation do not offer sufficient relief from intermittent claudication symptoms, intervention should be considered. Intermittent claudication symptoms that are mild probably do not warrant consideration for intervention with revascularization given the favorable natural history of the disease process as compared with the risks of intervention. In patients who experience lifestyle-limiting claudication despite conservative therapy, DSA with possible endovascular intervention such as angioplasty and/or stenting or surgical bypass should be considered. The decision to perform endovascular versus surgical revascularization is based mainly on the pattern and location of occlusive disease. In general, the more numerous, more severe, and longer the arterial lesions, the better the outcomes with surgical revascularization. Distinct criteria have been established by the TASC to differentiate which arterial occlusive lesions, are best treated with endovascular means and which are better served with surgical bypass.[10]

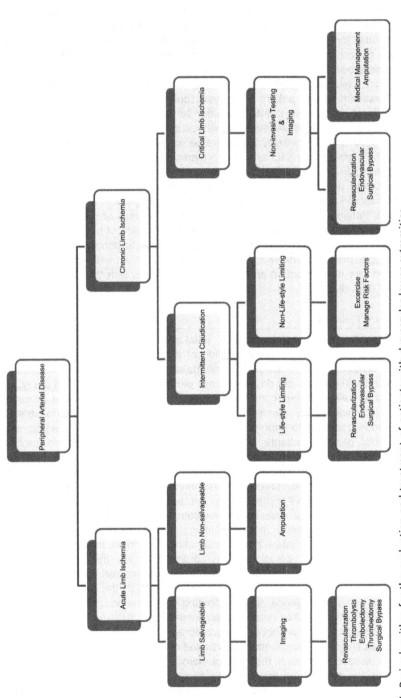

Fig. 6. Basic algorithm for the evaluation and treatment of patients with dysvascular lower extremities.

Critical Limb Ischemia

In the presence of ischemic rest pain or tissue loss, including ulceration and gangrene, predictors of nonhealing or progression to limb loss should be evaluated. These include nonpalpable pulses, decreased ABIs, and decreased toe pressures in the diabetic patient. If these factors predict nonhealing or elevated risk of limb loss, options for revascularization must be considered promptly.

The option of primary major amputation in the patient with CLI warrants discussion. In certain patients with CLI, major amputation (below-knee, knee disarticulation, or above-knee) may be a more appropriate option than efforts at limb revascularization. This group includes nonambulatory patients, patients with advanced tissue loss or gangrene that precludes foot salvage, patients in whom evaluation reveals nonrevascularizable occlusive disease, and patients with significant comorbidities or contraindications to leg revascularization efforts. Also, patients who have undergone multiple previous revascularization efforts that have failed may be better suited for amputation. The decision to perform amputation as a treatment option depends on the potential for healing, rehabilitation, and return of quality of life. Primary amputation tends to be an option in a minority of patients with CLI. It is crucial, even in patients who undergo primary amputation at the below-knee level or more proximally, that common femoral and profundus femoris artery inflow is assured for adequate healing. In patients with occlusive disease of the iliac, common femoral, or profunda femoris artery, revascularization to this level is usually required before major amputation to assure the highest chance of healing. One misconception is that superficial femoral artery and/or popliteal artery patency is required for healing of a below–knee level amputation. A below-knee amputation heals in most patients with superficial femoral artery occlusive disease in the setting of a patent common and profunda femoris artery, especially in the setting of chronic ischemia, which is often accompanied by multiple collateral vessels from the profunda femoris to the lower leg.

Options for Revascularization

Over the past decade, there have been significant trends toward the primary use of endovascular means of revascularization in the lower extremity. Formal recommendations for revascularization of the critically ischemic limb have been established by the TASC group.[9,10] Endovascular techniques should be primarily used to treat conditions in which the same level of symptomatic improvement will be obtained as when using open surgical techniques. The recommended treatment options for aortoiliac and femoral or popliteal lesions vary depending on the severity of the patient's disease. In general, endovascular procedures such as percutaneous balloon angioplasty and stenting are recommended for comparatively mild lesions, whereas surgical revascularization is recommended for patients with more severe occlusions or stenoses.

Endovascular Intervention

The imaging techniques described earlier play a crucial role in the decision-making process regarding revascularization of the ischemic extremity. Assuming that findings on noninvasive and invasive imaging predict low likelihood of healing, and therefore elevated risk of limb loss, revascularization should be considered. One advantage of DSA over noninvasive imaging modalities includes the option of performing therapeutic maneuvers at the same setting as the diagnostic procedure. The less severe the stenosis or occlusion the higher the likelihood that sufficient results can be obtained with percutaneous balloon angioplasty and/or stenting. Adjuvant techniques, such as laser atherectomy, rotational or excisional atherectomy, mechanical thrombolysis, cutting balloon technology, or cryoplasty balloon technology, may be used in combination with standard balloon angioplasty at the interventionalist's discretion.

Advances in endovascular technology have allowed for a wider applicability of these techniques to the ischemic extremity. Endovascular techniques have been demonstrated to be useful in treating even tibial vessel occlusive disease in the patient with CLI. The long-term patency of angioplasty of the infrapopliteal arteries is the subject of current investigation. One consideration to take into account is that even temporary improvement in arterial flow to the foot in patients with tissue loss or ulceration may be sufficient for wound healing (**Fig. 7**). When DSA is performed, the arterial flow from the aorta to the digital vessels of the foot may be evaluated in detail. It is generally considered a requirement that the limb has direct in-line flow to the foot via at least one of the 3 tibial vessels for the highest chance of wound healing. If direct in-line flow is absent, revascularization efforts should precede foot debridement or toe amputation.

When arterial flow to the foot is considered insufficient in the setting of CLI, endovascular treatment should be primarily considered. If this treatment is an option based on the anatomy of the occlusive disease, it may be performed during the same setting as the diagnostic arteriogram. Patients are typically loaded with clopidogrel and maintained on this antiplatelet agent for at least 30 days after an infrainguinal angioplasty procedure. The use of antiplatelet agents during this time may, however, require that foot debridement or minor amputation be performed while the patient is on these agents.

Surgical Revascularization

When PAD occlusive lesions are more extensive or efforts at endovascular intervention fails, surgical revascularization should be considered. Surgical options

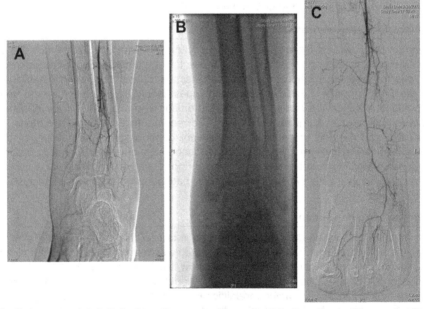

Fig. 7. Intra-arterial digital subtraction angiograms of a diabetic patient with a nonhealing toe ulcer. (*A*) Pretreatment angiogram showing minimal flow to foot. (*B*) Angioplasty balloon inflated. (*C*) Postangioplasty angiogram showing improved flow to the forefoot, which allowed the toe ulcer to heal.

are determined by 3 primary technical factors: inflow artery, outflow artery, and bypass conduit. In addition to these technical factors, patients' overall medical condition and their ability to withstand an operation must be taken into consideration. Preoperative cardiac assessment is generally made, and patients are medically optimized. Preoperative venous mapping is often performed to identify a suitable vein conduit for bypass grafting. Exceptions to this procedure include plans for aortobifemoral, axillofemoral, femoral-femoral, or iliofemoral artery bypass. For these procedures, prosthetic conduit is standardly used because it performs superior to vein conduit. Prosthetic bypass conduit options include polyester (Dacron) and polytetrafluoroethylene (PTFE). When femoral-popliteal artery bypass is planned to an above-knee target, prosthetic and vein conduits have been shown to have equivalent patency rates; therefore, choice of conduit is at the discretion of the surgeon. When veins are needed for infrainguinal bypass, options include the greater and lesser saphenous veins and the cephalic and basilic veins. Arm veins are used when leg veins are unavailable. Minimal vein diameter of 2 to 3 mm is generally preferred for adequate conduit. When no autologous vein is available for infrapopliteal bypass graft target, postoperative antiplatelet or anticoagulation therapy may be used in an effort to prolong patency of the prosthetic graft. Patency rates for prosthetic bypass grafts below the knee are inferior to those with autologous conduit.

A combined endovascular and open surgical technique may be used to improve the inflow for lower extremity bypass. One example of this technique is the use of iliac artery angioplasty and stenting to improve inflow for an infrainguinal bypass when both iliac and distal vessel disease are present. The goal of lower extremity revascularization in the patient with CLI is to establish in-line flow to the foot. Thus, bypass inflow and outflow arteries are chosen based on this goal. Bypass to vessels as distal as the plantar and tarsal arteries may be performed with encouraging results for foot salvage.[29]

Once surgical revascularization is performed, resolution of ischemic rest pain and healing of ulcerations is expected. When required, minor amputation may be performed and expected to heal. The patient who undergoes surgical bypass should also undergo a regimen of continued medical management of risk factors and bypass graft surveillance for life. Typical surveillance protocols include arterial duplex with ABI performed at 1, 3, 6, 12, 18, and 24 months postoperatively and annually thereafter. The long-term success of revascularization of the dysvascular limb highly depends on surveillance of the bypass graft and intervention with DSA and angioplasty if surveillance suggests the presence of graft stenosis of more than 50%.

SUMMARY

Given the aging population, the number of patients at risk for PAD and CLI will increase in the upcoming decade. Using a focused history and physical examination, along with a combination of noninvasive physiologic testing and noninvasive and invasive imaging modalities, one can accurately assess the location and physiologic effect of PAD. This assessment then allows the selection of the most appropriate treatment option for each patient. Treatment options may include exercise and risk-factor modification, amputation, and endovascular or surgical revascularization or a combination of both. A multispecialty approach to the patient with the dysvascular extremity is often required for the best clinical outcome.

REFERENCES

1. Selvin E, Erlinger TP. Prevalence of and risk factors for peripheral arterial disease in the United States: results from the National Health and Nutrition Examination Survey (1999–2000). Circulation 2004;110:738–43.
2. Hirsch A, Criqui M, Treat-Jacobson D, et al. Peripheral arterial disease detection, awareness and treatment in primary care. JAMA 2001;286(11):1317–24.
3. Norgren L, Hiatt WR, Dormandy JA, et al. TASC II working group. Inter-society consensus for the management of peripheral arterial disease (TASC II). J Vasc Surg 2007;45(Suppl S):S5–67.
4. Rosen AJ, DePalma RG. Risk factors in peripheral atherosclerosis. Arch Surg 1973;107(2):303–8.
5. Armstrong DG, Lavery LA. Diabetic foot ulcers: prevention, diagnosis and classification. Am Fam Physician 1998;57:1325–32.
6. Jones BA, Aly HM, Forsythe EA, et al. Phenotypic characterization of human smooth muscle cells derived from atherosclerotic tibial and peroneal arteries. J Vasc Surg 1996;24:883.
7. Weaver FA, Comerota AJ, Youngblood M, et al. Surgical revascularization versus thrombolysis for nonembolic lower extremity native artery occlusions: results of a prospective randomized trial. J Vasc Surg 1996;24:513–23.
8. Ouriel K, Veith FJ, Sasahara AA. A comparison of recombinanant urokinase with vascular surgery as initial treatment for acute arterial occlusion of the legs. Thrombolysis or Peripheral Arterial Surgery (TOPAS) Investigators. N Engl J Med 1998;338:1105–11.
9. Norgren L, Hiatt WR, Dormandy JA, et al. Inter-Society Consensus for the management of peripheral arterial disease (TASC II). J Vasc Surg 2007;33(S1): 1–75.
10. Dormandy JA, Rutherford RB. TransAtlantic inter-society consensus (TASC): management of peripheral arterial disease. J Vasc Surg 2000;31:S97.
11. Lundin M, Wiksten J, Perakyla T, et al. Distal pulse palpation: is it reliable? World J Surg 1999;23:252–5.
12. Boyko EJ, Afroni JF. Predictors of transcutaneous oxygen tension in the lower limbs of diabetic subjects. Diabet Med 1996;13:549–54.
13. Rooke TW, Osmundson PJ. The influence of age, sex, smoking and diabetes on lower limb transcutaneous oxygen tension in patients with arterial occlusive disease. Arch Intern Med 1990;150:129–32.
14. Ballard JL, Ede CC, Bunt TJ, et al. A prospective evaluation of transcutaneous oxygen measurements in the management of diabetic foot problems. J Vasc Surg 1995;22:485–90.
15. Apelqvist J, Castenfors J, Larsson J, et al. Prognostic value of systolic ankle and toe blood pressure levels in outcome of diabetic foot ulcer. Diabetes Care 1989; 12(6):373–8.
16. Vincent DG, Salles-Cunha SX, Bernhard VM, et al. Noninvasive assessment of toe systolic pressures with special reference to diabetes mellitus. J Cardiovasc Surg 1983;24:22–8.
17. Blakeman BM, Littooy FM, Baker WH. Intra-arterial digital subtraction angiography as a method to study peripheral vascular diseases. J Vasc Surg 1986;4: 168–73.
18. Aspelin P, Aubry P, Fransson SG, et al. Nephrotoxicity in high risk patients: Study of iso-osmolar and low-osmolar non-ionic contrast media. N Engl J Med 2003; 348:551–3.

19. Kuhn MJ, Chen N, Sahani DV, et al. The PREDICT study: a randomized double-blind comparison of contrast-induced nephropathy after low- or isoosmolar contrast agent exposure. AJR Am J Roentgenol 2008;191(1):151–7.
20. Solomon R, Werner C, Mann D, et al. Effects of saline, mannitol and furosemide on acute decreases in renal function by radiocontrast agents. N Engl J Med 1994; 331:1416–20.
21. Tepel M, Van der Giel M, Schwarfeld C, et al. Prevention of radiographic-contrast-agent-induced reductions in renal function by acetylcysteine. N Engl J Med 2000; 343:210–2.
22. Parfrey PS, Griffiths SM, Barret BJ, et al. Contrast material-induced renal failure in patients with diabetes mellitus, renal insufficiency, or both: a prospective controlled study. N Engl J Med 1989;320:143.
23. Lawrence JA, Kim D, Kent KC, et al. Lower extremity spiral CT angiography versus catheter angiography. Radiology 1995;194:903–8.
24. Ota H, Takase K, Igarashi K, et al. MDCT compared with digital subtraction angiography for assessment of lower extremity arterial occlusive disease: importance of reviewing cross-sectional images. AJR Am J Roentgenol 2004;182(1):201–9.
25. Koelemay MJ, Lijmer JG, Stoker J, et al. Magnetic resonance angiography for the evaluation of lower extremity arterial disease. JAMA 2001;285(10):1338–45.
26. Cambria RP, Kaufman JA, L'Italien GJ, et al. Magnetic resonance angiography in the management of lower extremity arterial occlusive disease: a prospective study. J Vasc Surg 1997;25(2):380–9.
27. CAPRIE Steering Committee. A randomized, blinded trial of clopidogrel versus aspirin in patients at risk of ischemic events (CAPRIE). Lancet 1996;348:1329–39.
28. Nehler MR, Hiatt WR. Exercise therapy for claudication. Ann Vasc Surg 1999;13: 109–14.
29. Hughes K, Domenig CM, Hamdan AD, et al. Bypass to plantar and tarsal arteries: an acceptable approach to limb salvage. J Vasc Surg 2004;40:1149–57.

Bone and Wound Healing in the Diabetic Patient

Siddhant K. Mehta, Eric A. Breitbart, MD,
Wayne S. Berberian, MD, Frank A. Liporace, MD,
Sheldon S. Lin, MD*

KEYWORDS

- Bone healing • Wound healing • Diabetes mellitus
- Foot and ankle surgery

Diabetes mellitus (DM) is a systemic disease that results from the inability to maintain glucose homeostasis. The clinical importance of DM in the United States cannot be overstated, with more than 23 million people affected and an additional 1.6 million new cases diagnosed each year.[1,2] Management of musculoskeletal pathology in diabetic patients represents a significant challenge to the orthopedic surgeon. DM has a known profound deleterious effect on bone and soft tissue healing, thus yielding a high rate of delayed union or nonunion and wound complications in patients sustaining traumatic injury (ie, fracture) or undergoing elective surgery (ie, arthrodesis).[3–9]

The pathophysiology of DM has been well described. With prolonged periods of hyperglycemia secondary to alterations in insulin levels or insulin receptor affinity, the production of advanced glycation end products (AGEs) ensues. Accumulation of AGEs in vascular tissues causes alteration of the function of endothelial cells, smooth muscle cells, and macrophages, and further leads to the conventional complications associated with DM, including micro- and macroangiopathy. The resulting ischemia, coupled with altered cellular function, creates an unfavorable environment for the appropriate regeneration of bone and soft tissue in response to injury.

In an effort to augment healing in patients with DM, several management options, both intraoperative and perioperative, have been explored. Conventional surgical fixation techniques have been modified to improve osseous repair in diabetic patients. Recent interest has focused on the local application of various biologic agents to provide an immediate, high-dose delivery of essential growth factors to promote healing at the surgical site in high-risk patients.[3,10–14] Perioperatively, enhanced glucose control

No financial disclosures.
Department of Orthopaedics, University of Medicine and Dentistry of New Jersey, New Jersey Medical School, 90 Bergen Street, Doctor's Office Clinic, Suite 7300, Newark, NJ 07103, USA
* Corresponding author.
E-mail address: linss@umdnj.edu

and oxygen supplementation can improve union rates in diabetic patients. In addition, biophysical stimulation methods, namely low-intensity pulsed ultrasonography (LIPUS)[15–17] and electrical bone stimulation devices,[18] have been investigated, yielding promising results with their utility in the postoperative period for high-risk patients.

This article aims to describe the impact of DM on bone and soft tissue healing, and identify the available treatment modalities that can potentially enhance osseous healing and reduce wound complication rates to further improve clinical outcomes in diabetic patients undergoing foot and ankle surgery.

CLINICAL CONSIDERATIONS

A multitude of risk factors are known to play a role in impaired bone and soft tissue healing, including age, smoking, immunosuppression, peripheral vascular disease, medications, and certain systemic diseases.[19] Among this array of factors, DM is a systemic disease that has profound unfavorable effects on bone and soft tissue regeneration, namely delayed osseous healing and impaired wound healing (**Fig. 1**).

Impaired Osseous Healing

Despite ongoing advances in orthopedics to enhance bone healing, about 10% of the 6 million annual fractures still develop delayed union or nonunion.[20] Furthermore, 20% to 40% of all ankle arthrodeses, especially in high-risk patients, result in delayed union or nonunion.[6–9,21] Similarly, in failed syndesmotic fusion for Agility ankle replacement, osteolysis and component loosening are known complications of total ankle arthroplasty from the delayed union.[22] DM is among the various factors that can be attributed to these complications, and its deleterious effect on bone healing (**Fig. 2**) has been well described in animal models.[23–26] To better recognize the impact of DM on osseous healing in foot and ankle surgery, one may review the clinical studies about acute fractures[4,5] and arthrodesis.[3,6–9]

In an early case report, Cozen[4] first observed the effect of DM on healing time for lower extremity fractures in 9 consecutive diabetic patients. A prolonged time to achieve union was demonstrated in each diabetic case when compared with 9 control cases of matched age and fractures. Loder[5] further investigated healing time in a retrospective review of 31 fractures in 28 diabetic patients sustaining closed lower extremity fractures when compared with expected healing time (as determined by a review of the literature) for the same fracture type and treatment method in the general population. In this study, the union time in diabetic patients was 163% that of the control population. In addition, displaced fractures and those fractures repaired by open reduction resulted in prolonged union time (187% and 186%, respectively) when compared with nondisplaced fractures and treatment with closed reduction, respectively. In light of these findings, Cozen and Loder concluded that DM significantly impaired fracture healing.

A more recent study by Boddenberg[27] reviewed the literature and described results of a case series of 80 patients to assess healing time in diabetic versus nondiabetic patients sustaining fractures of the foot (35 diabetic patients with neuropathic Charcot fractures) and ankle (28 diabetic patients, 17 nondiabetic patients). In contrast to findings by previous investigators, this study demonstrated only a slight increase in healing time, with a median of 3.5 months in diabetic patients compared with 3 months in nondiabetic patients.

Several investigators have reported the outcome of foot and/or ankle arthrodesis in patients with DM.[3,6–9] In a prospective clinical study, Papa and colleagues[6] described the results of open reduction and arthrodesis in 29 patients with diabetic neuropathic

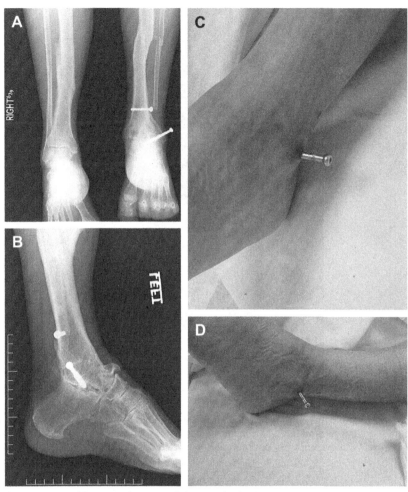

Fig. 1. A 53-year-old man with type 1 diabetes who had an attempted ankle fusion 3 years previously. Radiographs at 1 year after surgery demonstrate nonunion with failure of hardware (ie, screw backing out) as seen on anteroposterior (A) and lateral (B) views of the ankle. Clinical pictures (C, D) at 2 years after surgery demonstrate exposed hardware with cellulitis.

arthropathy. Depending on the joints involved, the appropriate joint arthrodesis was performed (tibiocalcaneal, tibiotalar, tibio-talo-calcaneal, pantalar, or triple arthrodesis), and the clinical outcome in these patients was evaluated. Solid fusion failed to develop in 10 of the 29 patients (34.5%) in whom pseudoarthrosis was present. A clinically stable pseudoarthrosis, with respect to the ability to stand and walk, was present in 7 of the 10 patients. However, 3 patients presented with an unstable pseudoarthrosis that resulted in nonunion requiring amputation, repeat operation (which achieved a stable pseudoarthrosis), or the use of a permanent ankle-foot orthotic for weight bearing and/or walking. In addition, 2 of the 28 cases developed malunion associated with deformities.

Similarly, a large retrospective review by Perlman and Thordarson[7] studied the outcome of 88 ankle fusions in patients, with 67 described as having "complete"

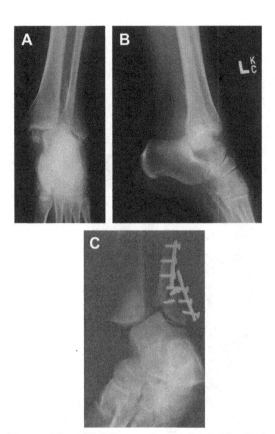

Fig. 2. A 42-year-old man with type 1 diabetes who sustained a bimalleolar equivalent ankle fracture requiring surgical intervention, as seen on anteroposterior (*A*) and lateral (*B*) views of the ankle, with evidence of nonunion and hardware failure (*C*) 6 months after surgery.

assessment by preoperative, intraoperative, and postoperative radiographs. One significant risk factor that the investigators found to lead to nonunion was those patients who sustained an "open fracture." Additional risk factors were analyzed, including presence of DM, and 3 of 8 diabetic patients (38%) developed nonunion compared with 14 of 51 nondiabetic patients (27%). Although statistical significance was not reached with respect to DM as a risk factor for nonunion attributable to low sample size, a trend regarding the negative impact of DM on osseous healing was noted.

Chahal and colleagues[3] conducted a retrospective case series to assess the outcome of subtalar arthrodesis in 88 patients with primary or secondary osteoarthritis. Radiological and functional outcomes were evaluated via radiographs (lateral foot; oblique and axial hindfoot views) and questionnaires (AAOS Foot and Ankle Outcome Instrument and Short Musculoskeletal Function Assessment), respectively, to determine successful union and overall function, pain, and patient satisfaction. After adjusting for age and sex, the results of this study showed that the likelihood of varus malunion in diabetic patients (n = 9) was 18.7 times higher than that in nondiabetic patients ($P<.05$). Furthermore, diabetic patients had significantly poorer functional outcomes when compared with the other patients in this study.

The described clinical observations clearly implicate that DM significantly impedes osseous healing in both fracture repair and arthrodesis, suggesting that adequate blood glucose control may improve clinical outcomes in diabetic patients. However, the need exists for prospective controlled clinical trials with adequate sample sizes to definitively determine the effect of DM on foot and ankle osseous healing.

Impaired Wound Healing

Fractures about the ankle comprise the most common type of injury treated by orthopedic surgeons, with an annual incidence of 250,000 cases.[28] Because the ankle is enveloped by such a limited amount of soft tissue, significant soft tissue and wound complications often occur after surgical treatment (**Figs. 3** and **4**). Therefore, a delay in definitive operative treatment has been used to allow soft tissue swelling to decrease and healing to begin.[29,30] However, soft tissue complications after operative management of ankle fractures still range from 2% to 5.3% to 8.3% to 60% in diabetic patients.[28,31–33]

In 1985, investigators at the Centers for Disease Control developed a predictive score in a study of 120,000 patients to classify those at risk for developing postoperative wound infections.[34] The Study on the Effect of Nosocomial Infection Control (SENIC) assigned 1 point each to 4 "effectors" of wound infection development. The 4 variables included, in order of importance, (1) abdominal site of surgery, (2) contaminated or dirty wound, (3) more than 2 hours of operative time, and (4) 3 or more

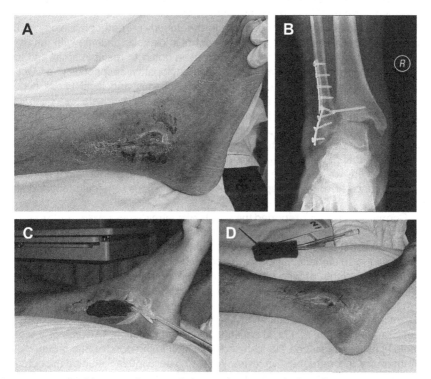

Fig. 3. A 53-year-old man with type 1 diabetes who sustained a bimalleolar equivalent ankle fracture requiring surgical intervention complicated by wound dehiscence and hardware failure (*A*, *B*). A KCI wound VAC (vacuum-assisted closure; Kinetic Concepts, Inc, San Antonio, TX, USA) was placed (*C*), with signs of clinical improvement at 6 days after VAC placement (*D*).

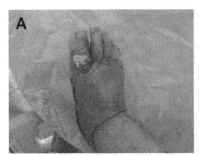 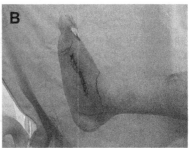

Fig. 4. A 47-year-old man with type 1 diabetes who was admitted for intravenous antibiotics for the diagnosis of cellulitis 1 week after a midfoot fusion for Charcot arthropathy. The extent of the cellulitis was marked at the time of admission (*A, B*).

comorbid diagnoses (eg, DM, hypertension, cardiac, pulmonary, or other systemic diseases). The possible score ranges were 0 to 4, with a score of 0 predictive of an infection rate less than 1% and a score of 4 predictive of a 24% to 27% infection rate. Other effectors of surgical wound infections have also been identified, including low pH and uncontrolled glucose,[35] hypoperfusion,[36,37] hypothermia,[35] and pain.[38] The common theme among the latter 3 effectors is the association of decreased subcutaneous oxygen tension and tissue hypoxia.[35–38]

Hyperglycemia is the primary concern in the underlying pathophysiology of DM. Failure to appropriately achieve glycemic control in diabetic patients with the use of oral hypoglycemic agents and/or insulin has been noted to result in small and large vessel pathology (microangiopathy and macroangiopathy, respectively) as well as endothelial cellular dysfunction. Consequently, ischemia and local tissue hypoxia develop, and collagen production is severely impaired as fibroblasts lose their ability to migrate and proliferate under hypoxic conditions. In addition, the ischemic environment results in an increased susceptibility to infection, which may further complicate the healing process secondary to the release of various bacterial enzymes and metalloproteinases that have a degradative effect on fibrin and numerous growth factors. Hence, impaired wound healing is a significant problem in patients with uncontrolled DM, as evidenced by several reported clinical observations regarding foot and ankle surgery.

McCormack and Leith[39] reported the results of a retrospective case-control study in which they compared the outcomes of 26 diabetic patients sustaining ankle fractures with 26 nondiabetic controls, matched for patient age, fracture type, and treating surgeon. Of the 19 diabetic patients who received operative intervention, 5 developed wound complications, of whom 2 developed septic arthritis and 2 developed deep infection requiring amputation, eventually leading to death.

Flynn and colleagues[40] retrospectively studied infection rates in patients with closed ankle fractures, comparing diabetic patients with nondiabetic patients. Among the diabetic group, 8 of the 25 (32%) patients developed infection, whereas only 6 of 68 patients (8.8%) experienced the same complication in the nondiabetic group.

Furthermore, in a retrospective review White and colleagues[41] studied the outcome of 14 open ankle fractures in 13 patients with DM. Wound complications were observed in 9 of the 14 fractures, 6 of which required below-knee amputation.

In a more recent, larger clinical retrospective case series, Costigan and colleagues[42] reviewed outcomes in diabetic patients sustaining unstable ankle fractures who were managed operatively with open reduction and internal fixation. Infection was observed in 10 of the 84 patients (11.9%), of whom 2 required below-the-knee amputation. In addition, among various patient variables, peripheral vascular disease and peripheral neuropathy were identified as significant risk factors (P<.0001) for developing complications, as evidenced by complication rates of 83.3% and 91.6%, respectively.

Kline and colleagues[43] recently reported the early complications following operative management of pilon fractures. In this retrospective study, the outcomes of surgery (staged open reduction and internal fixation, external fixation, or primary fusion) for 14 fractures in 13 diabetic patients and 69 fractures in 68 nondiabetic patients were reviewed. Among the 14 diabetic fractures, 4 developed superficial infection while 6 developed deep infection, with an overall infection rate of 71.4% compared with 19% in the nondiabetic group.

Similarly, Wukich[44] recently performed a retrospective review of 1000 consecutive foot and ankle surgical cases to assess infection rates in patients with and without DM. Patients with obvious preoperative infection were excluded from the study. Postoperative infection was defined to occur within 30 days of surgery, or up to 30 days after removal of hardware in patients who had external fixation. Infections were characterized to be mild (<2-cm erythema receiving outpatient antibiotic treatment) or severe (>2-cm erythema receiving inpatient intravenous antibiotics and/or surgical incision and draining). An overall infection rate of 4.8% was reported; 13.2% of the diabetic patient population demonstrated infection, whereas only 2.8% of the nondiabetic control group demonstrated the same. In addition, significant correlation with increased infection rates was shown to be associated with peripheral neuropathy, history of a previous ulcer, and external fixation, as determined by a multivariate analysis in this study. Furthermore, a secondary analysis compared infection rates among nondiabetic patients, patients with uncomplicated diabetes without end organ complications, and patients with complicated diabetes with end organ damage. Results showed that infection rate was highest in the complicated diabetes group (16.7%), with lower infection rates in the uncomplicated diabetic and nondiabetic groups (3.5% and 1.8%, respectively).

While further investigation through prospective clinical studies is warranted, these clinical series reveal that impaired wound healing and an increased susceptibility to infection are associated with DM and, therefore, the management of diabetic patients undergoing foot and ankle surgery is an exceptionally challenging endeavor.

INTRAOPERATIVE MANAGEMENT

For the successful management of diabetic patients requiring foot and ankle surgery, special attention must be given to appropriate surgical fixation techniques, which can reduce the risk of soft tissue complications and delayed osseous healing associated with DM. With the recent development of certain techniques to supplement standard ankle fixation, namely supplementary K-wires in plated fibulas, locked plating, and the use of tetra-cortical fibula-to-tibia screw fixation, and the local application of certain biologic adjuncts to facilitate and further enhance osseous healing, a reduction in complications in patients with DM can be achieved.

Fixation Techniques

Over the years, surgeons have developed several techniques to minimize complications associated with osteopenic bone, commonly seen with diabetic ankle fractures. Operatively indicated fractures in diabetic patients require very rigid fixation to avoid loss of reduction. In addition, the importance of soft tissue stabilization must be considered.

Bibbo and colleagues[31] have emphasized the importance of a protocol to appropriately manage patients with ankle fractures, involving initially a timely reduction and splinting to reduce soft tissue trauma, followed by surgical intervention after edema resolves and medical status is optimized. An external fixator may be necessary to maintain reduction pending soft tissue stabilization, and can be combined with internal fixation based on the ultimate condition of the soft tissue envelope.[31,45] External fixation may be either the first part of a staged reconstruction or a definitive treatment if severe concomitant soft tissue injury is present.

Osteopenia or osteoporosis is a frequent concern in the management of diabetic patients, and supplementation to standard ankle fixation in these patients is often necessary. Koval and colleagues[46] described a technique for superior screw purchase during fibula plate fixation in osteoporotic bone to minimize loss of reduction and malunion (**Fig. 5**). First, 1.6-mm K-wires are placed across a reduced distal fibula fracture in a retrograde manner, with penetration of the medial fibular cortex in the proximal fragment. Next, a precontoured one-third tubular plate is fixed to the lateral aspect of the fibula with screws interdigitating with the intramedullary retrograde K-wires. In their retrospective study, Koval and colleagues[46] described 19 patients who underwent this technique, all of whom went on to achieve union without loss of reduction. At a mean follow-up of 15.4 months, 17 of 19 patients (89%) had no pain, slight pain, or mild pain. In conjunction with the clinical series, biomechanical testing in cadaver models demonstrated this construct to be superior to standard fixation with tubular plate alone, as specimens augmented with K-wires had 81% greater resistance to bending and twice the resistance to motion during torsional testing.[46]

To further enhance fixation stiffness on the augmented K-wire model, Schon and Marks[45] described the use of multiple tetra-cortical fibula-to-tibia screws to provide fixation through the one-third tubular plate in the proximal fibula fragment (**Fig. 6**).[45,47] In comparison with the intramedullary K-wire augmented fixation, biomechanical testing of a similar construct with the addition of 3 tetra-cortical syndesmotic screws was shown to be significantly stiffer in resisting axial and external rotation loads.[47] Moreover, a recent case series by Perry and colleagues[48] described the outcomes in 6 patients with failed neuropathic ankle fractures who underwent a similar technique with the addition of a 4.5-mm dynamic compression plate and multiple 4.5-mm tetra-cortical syndesmotic screws. At final follow-up, all patients were satisfied with their results.[48] The utility of fibula-to-tibia tetra-cortical screws has been suggested to alter the biomechanics of the ankle by changing the stiffness of the syndesmosis, specifically decreasing tibiotalar external rotation and anterior-posterior drawer in plantar flexion. Although hardware failure (ie, screw breakage) is a major concern when using this technique,[49] it has not been shown to be a significant problem clinically, because ambulation progressively restores motion between the tibia and fibula despite fixation, as evidenced by lysis around the syndesmotic screws. Moreover, in certain fracture patterns with significant fibular comminution and degeneration at the tibiofibular joint, it is difficult to achieve syndesmotic screw fixation. In such cases, multiple screw fixation ensures restoration of fibular length and maintenance of the tibia-fibula relationship.

In addition, a retrospective review by Jani and colleagues[50] described retrograde transcalcaneal-talar-tibial fixation with Steinmann pins or screws (**Fig. 7**) and prolonged, protected weight bearing to supplement standard techniques of open reduction and internal fixation in 15 diabetic neuropathic patients with unstable ankle fractures. In contrast to previously reported complication rates of between 30% and

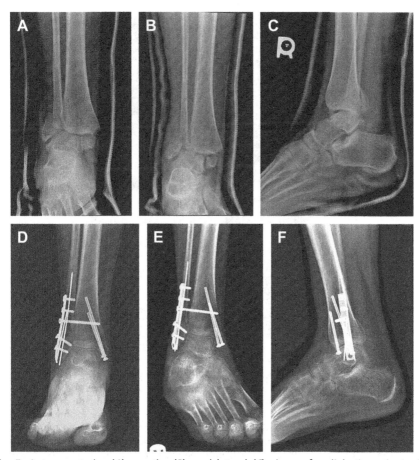

Fig. 5. Anteroposterior (A), mortise (B), and lateral (C) views of a diabetic patient with a right bimalleolar ankle fracture with a syndesmotic injury. Ankle series after fixation (D, E, F), showing placement of 3 retrograde 1.6-mm K-wires across the fibula fracture to enhance screw purchase. (From Chaudhary SB, Liporace FA, Gandhi A, et al. Complications of ankle fracture in patients with diabetes. J Am Acad Orthop Surg 2008;16(3):166; with permission. Copyright © 2008 American Academy of Orthopedic Surgeons.)

43% for diabetic patients with and without neuropathy, this study reported lower major complication rates for all fractures (25%) and closed fractures (23%) in diabetic neuropathic patients. A stable ankle capable of weight bearing was demonstrated in 13 of 15 patients (87%) with the transarticular fixation method described in conjunction with prolonged, protected weight bearing.

Another potential technique to enhance surgical fixation for high-risk patients was introduced using locked plating (Fig. 8). With this method, screws are locked in the plate at a fixed angle, minimizing the compressive forces exerted by the plate on the bone. Fixed-angle screws do not rely on friction between the plate and bone; therefore in order for hardware failure to occur, "cutting out" all of the points of fixation on one side of the fracture is required, as opposed to loosening of individual screws as is seen with traditional plating. Recent biomechanical studies have shown that when subjected to cyclical loading, locked-plate fixation can better retain its original

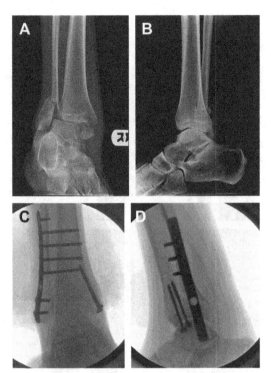

Fig. 6. An attempted mortise (*A*) and lateral (*B*) view of a 19-year-old type I diabetic patient status post motor vehicle accident with a right bimalleolar ankle fracture and a syndesmotic injury. Postfixation mortise (*C*) and lateral (*D*) views. This patient with brittle diabetes underwent locked plate fixation with 4 tetra-cortical syndesmotic screws for his injury complex. The medial side was fixed with 2 standard partially threaded screws. (*From* Chaudhary SB, Liporace FA, Gandhi A, et al. Complications of ankle fracture in patients with diabetes. J Am Acad Orthop Surg 2008;16(3):167; with permission. Copyright © 2008 American Academy of Orthopedic Surgeons.)

stiffness compared with traditional plating.[51,52] However, further prospective clinical studies are needed to evaluate long-term outcomes of ankle fractures managed with locked plating.

Orthobiologics

While appropriate surgical fixation is essential when performing foot and ankle trauma or elective surgery on diabetic patients, the need to overcome the impaired osseous healing and soft tissue regeneration associated with DM is apparent. In an effort to address this concern several biologic agents, both autologous and recombinant, have been explored to further reduce complication rates and improve clinical outcomes in this high-risk patient population. Collectively known as orthobiologics, these agents consist of various growth factors and secretory proteins that have been shown to be essential during the healing process. Platelet-rich plasma (PRP) and bone morphogenetic proteins (BMPs) are among the orthobiologics that have gained recent interest, showing promising results when applied locally at the surgical site in various orthopedic applications, including foot and ankle surgery, to facilitate management in high-risk patients (**Figs. 9** and **10**).

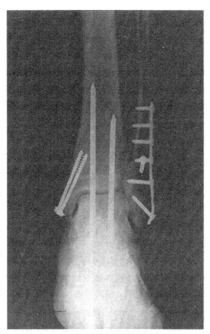

Fig. 7. Example of retrograde transcalcaneal-talar-tibial fixation with Steinmann pins and screws in a high-risk ankle fracture in a neuropathic diabetic patient.

Platelet-rich plasma

PRP is derived from autologous blood and contains a concentrated volume of platelets, as well as growth factors and bioactive proteins that influence healing of musculoskeletal tissues. These growth factors, which play a role in various stages of osseous and soft tissue healing, include platelet-derived growth factor (PDGF), transforming growth factor (TGF), insulin-like growth factor (IGF), vascular endothelial growth factor (VEGF), and epidermal growth factor (EGF).[53,54]

Although several scientific studies have described a favorable effect of PRP on bone and soft tissue healing, there are limited data currently available that definitively describe the role of the clinical application of PRP on diabetic patients undergoing foot and ankle surgery. Several investigators have proposed that PRP can serve as a safe adjunct with significant augmentation of osseous healing, namely fusion, when applied locally, especially in high-risk patients.

Gandhi and colleagues[55] investigated the effect of PRP in 9 patients who sustained foot and ankle fractures complicated by nonunion in an early prospective preliminary study. Patients diagnosed with nonunion for a minimum duration of 4 months (up to 10 months) following their initial fracture repair underwent a revision operation consisting of a combination of PRP and autogenous bone graft applied to the nonunion site using standard fixation techniques. Union was achieved at a mean of 60 days after revision surgery with PRP and autogenous bone graft in all patients. Investigators also quantified growth factor concentrations at the surgical site within the fracture hematoma in patients with and without nonunion. A significant reduction in levels of PDGF and TGF-β was noted locally at the fracture site in patients with nonunion versus fresh fracture, whereas plasma levels of these growth factors remained consistent.

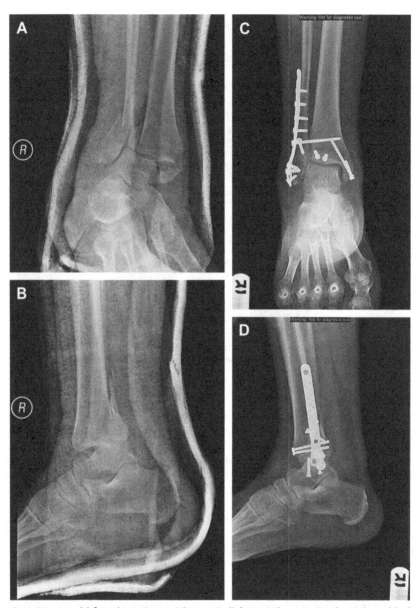

Fig. 8. A 51-year-old female patient with type 2 diabetes who sustained a right ankle fracture dislocation as seen on anteroposterior (A) and lateral (B) views of the ankle. She underwent definitive fixation with a fibular locking plate and syndesmotic screw owing to her osteopenia, as shown on postoperative anteroposterior (C) and lateral (D) views of the ankle.

In a prospective evidence-based study, Gandhi and colleagues[54] demonstrated the use of PRP in high-risk patients undergoing elective foot and ankle surgery. Patients enrolled in this study were identified to have at least 1 risk factor for poor or delayed osseous healing. After the application of PRP alone, or in combination with bone graft

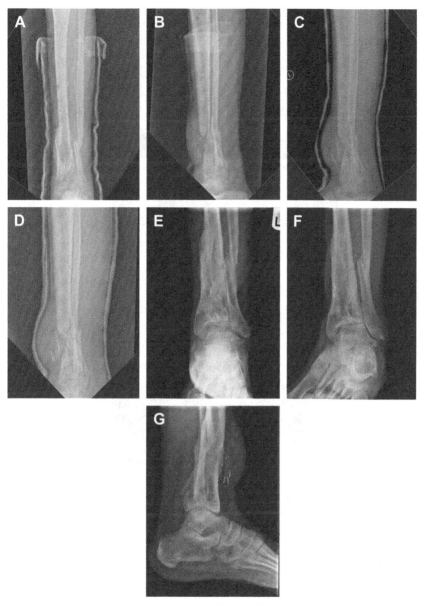

Fig. 9. Preoperative anteroposterior (*A*) and lateral (*B*) views of the left ankle demonstrating distal tibial nonunion. Fourteen days postoperative bone grafting with PRP demonstrates early callus formation (*C*); 28 days postoperative bone grafting with PRP demonstrates more callus formation (*D*); 2-year follow-up anteroposterior (*E*), mortise (*F*), and lateral (*G*) views of the left ankle demonstrate healed nonunion.

(if bony defect was present or correction of alignment was necessary) at the site of surgical intervention for various pathologies involving the hindfoot, forefoot, or ankle, 62 high-risk patients (encompassing 123 operative procedures) were observed for a period of 6 months. Overall, a 94% union rate was achieved at a mean of

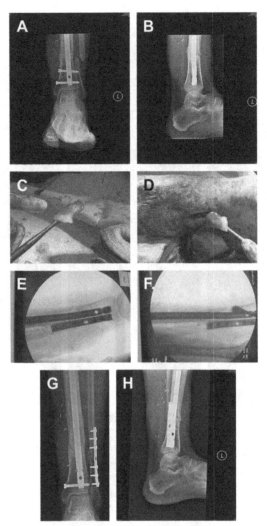

Fig. 10. A 43-year-old diabetic man who underwent open reduction and internal fixation (ORIF) of the left open tibia-fibula fracture with a free flap. The patient presented with a malunion/nonunion at 1 year post surgery, as seen on anteroposterior (A) and lateral (B) views of the ankle. Definitive treatment included plating of the fibula with percutaneous placement of rhBMP-2 on an absorbable collagen sponge (C, D, E, F). Follow-up films demonstrate union of the tibia and fibula at 6 months after revision surgery, as seen on anteroposterior (G) and lateral (H) views of the ankle.

41 days. Patients treated with PRP alone demonstrated a mean time of 40 days to achieve union, whereas a mean of 45 days was required to achieve union in patients who received bone graft in addition to PRP. Nonetheless, the conclusion drawn by the investigators supported the use of PRP as an adjunct to facilitate healing in high-risk elective foot and ankle surgery to reduce complication rates.

The utility of PRP for ankle syndesmotic fusion in total ankle replacement (TAR) has also been recently explored. Barrow and Pomeroy[56] analyzed the effect of PRP-augmented bone grafting on syndesmotic fusion rates in patients receiving an Agility

TAR. In this study, 20 consecutive patients previously diagnosed with posttraumatic arthritis, rheumatoid arthritis, or osteoarthritis underwent TAR after failure of at least 6 months of conservative management. Symphony PCS autologous platelet concentrate (Depuy Corp, Warsaw, IN) was sprayed on the bone surfaces of the syndesmosis, on the cut surfaces of the distal tibia and talus, and over the porous coating of the ankle prosthesis. PRP was also mixed with local autograft derived from resected bone, which was packed in the distal tibiofibular joint after insertion of the TAR components. Within 6 months, successful fusion of the syndesmosis occurred in all 20 cases, as compared with distal tibiofibular joint fusion rates of 62% to 82% at 6 months previously reported by other investigators.[57,58] Similarly, Coetzee and colleagues[22] assessed fusion rates in 66 patients receiving PRP-augmented bone grafting of the ankle syndesmosis during TAR in comparison with 114 historical controls with non-PRP–augmented bone grafting. On radiographic evaluation, a statistically significant difference was observed with respect to fusion rates at 8-week and 12-week time points between the control group (61.4% and 73.6%, respectively) and study group (76% and 93.9%, respectively). A significantly reduced number of delayed unions and nonunions in the study group was also observed.

More recently, in a prospective case series, Pinzur[59] studied the effects of PRP and bone marrow aspirate in high-risk patients with Charcot arthropathy of the foot. In this study, 44 diabetic patients (46 feet) at high risk for poor clinical outcome with conventional surgery underwent surgical correction for their deformities, during which a static external fixator was applied to maintain postoperative surgical correction, followed by the injection of freshly prepared PRP and bone marrow aspirate into the fusion site before wound closure. Partial weight bearing was allowed for 8 weeks, after which the external fixator was removed, and a total contact cast was placed for 4 to 6 weeks. Of all fusion sites, 91.3% (n = 46) demonstrated radiographic evidence of union at 16 weeks after surgery. In addition, patients were able to ambulate using therapeutic footwear, indicating clinically acceptable results.

Bone morphogenetic proteins

BMPs are the key modulators of osteoprogenitor and mesenchymal cells during osseous healing. There have been more than 20 BMPs identified thus far, all of which belong to the TGF-β superfamily of proteins, with the exception of BMP-1. The regulatory role of BMPs in the differentiation and proliferation of mesenchymal stem cell into cartilage and bone-forming cells during osseous healing has been studied.[60] New bone formation occurs in response to the stimulatory effect of BMPs on endochondral ossification and, in high concentrations, on intramembranous ossification.[61] BMP-2, BMP-4, and BMP-7 have been shown to have to have prominent roles in new bone formation.[14] With recent advances in molecular biology, genetic engineering techniques have enabled the manufacture of synthetic growth factors, such as recombinant human bone morphogenetic proteins (rhBMPs), for experimental and clinical applications. At this time, rhBMP-2 and rhBMP-7 are the only BMPs commercially available. The Food and Drug Administration (FDA) approved rhBMP-2 for clinical use in only certain orthopedic applications (open tibia fracture and posterior lumbar fusion), and rhBMP-7 as humanitarian device exemption for failed treated tibia nonunions.[62]

A few clinical studies have reported on the successful use of rhBMP-2 in foot and ankle surgery. Bibbo and Haskell[63] conducted the first prospective study investigating the effect of rhBMP-2 in complex foot and ankle arthrodesis. In 45 procedures, the mean time to achieve union was reported to be 10 weeks (range 4–30 weeks), whereas wound complications were observed in only 2 patients. A retrospective analysis was recently performed by Bibbo and colleagues[64] to follow up their initial case series with a study of 69 high-risk patients (112 procedures) undergoing foot and ankle arthrodesis with the local application of rhBMP-2 at the fusion site. These patients were categorized as high risk based on risk factors for poor bone healing including DM, high-energy injury, and immunosuppression. Successful union was achieved in 108 of the 112 fusion sites (96.4%), with a mean time of 11 weeks to achieve union. Furthermore, no significant difference in union rates was seen among the various different sites of fusion. Only 3 of the 69 patients (4.3%) developed wound complications, which were successfully treated with appropriate local wound care and antibiotics.

PERIOPERATIVE MANAGEMENT

Perioperative planning and management are important when treating high-risk patients, such as persons with diabetes, for foot and ankle pathology. The administration of supplementary oxygen and appropriate glucose control has been shown to reduce infection rates and wound complications. In addition, osseous healing may be accelerated with the use of biophysical stimulation in the postoperative period. Although the need exists for prospective clinical data to definitively describe the effect of each of these perioperative considerations on diabetic bone and wound healing, several clinical observations have described their potential benefits.

Oxygen

Tissue hypoxia, by definition, implies a local oxygen deficiency. One clinical entity, chronic granulomatous disease, occurs secondary to a genetic absence of a nicotinamide adenine dinucleotide phosphate (NADPH)-oxidase and is manifested by repeated infections despite antibiotics. This clinical entity demonstrates the key role of oxygen and NADPH-oxidase, with the link between ineffective bacterial killing and infection.[35] The primary mechanism of bacterial killing occurs during phagocytosis and is mediated by the NADPH-linked oxidase. Within the phagosome, NADPH-oxidase uses oxygen as a substrate, with NADPH as a cofactor, to produce superoxide (free radical) and other oxidants (with H_2O_2) that have bactericidal properties.[65] Therefore, insufficient levels of oxygen will significantly inhibit the leukocyte bactericidal activity.

Allen and colleagues[35] have analyzed this complex relationship of human neutrophils, oxygen consumption, and superoxide production under conditions of varying oxygen pressures (Po_2), pH values, temperatures, and glucose concentrations. The investigators found that half-maximal oxidant production occurred in the Po_2 range of 45 to 80 mm Hg and that maximal production occurred at Po_2 higher than 300 mm Hg. It was also noted that oxidant generation, to a lesser extent, was also dependent on pH, temperature, and glucose levels.

Hopf and colleagues[66] applied Allen's work to a prospective study in which tissue Po_2 was measured in 130 general surgical patients and the rates of wound infections were observed. Tissue Po_2 was measured at a baseline fraction of inspired oxygen (Fio_2) (room air or percentage of Fio_2 necessary to keep oxygen saturation at 90%–96%) and at a maximal Fio_2 (%Fio_2 doubled the baseline amount). Tissue Po_2 in patients after surgery (49 mm Hg O_2 baseline, 69 mm Hg O_2 maximal) was found to be lower than that of healthy, nonoperative controls (65 mm Hg O_2 baseline and 130 mm Hg O_2 maximal). Hopf and colleagues[66] hypothesized that subcutaneous wound oxygen tension had an inverse correlation with the development of postoperative wound infections. Using the aforementioned SENIC score as a gold standard, Hopf and colleagues[66] concluded that low subcutaneous wound Po_2 is a stronger predictor of development of surgical wound infections (43% infection prediction in the highest risk group vs SENIC's 27% prediction; $P<.05$).

Other work by Chang and colleagues[36] also documented postoperative surgical wound hypoxia in a study of 33 patients. The investigators noted a biphasic relationship between arterial (Pao_2) and tissue Po_2, likely curvilinear at the lower range of Pao_2 and rising linearly as Pao_2 increases, even above the point of full saturation of hemoglobin. Furthermore, they noted the difficulty in determining tissue hypoxia by routine clinical parameters (eg, oxygen saturation, arterial blood gas, signs of euvolemia).

In a larger prospective, double-blind series, Greif and colleagues[67] studied 500 patients undergoing elective colon resection who were randomized to receive 30% or 80% supplemental oxygen during the perioperative period. The investigators hypothesized that the 80% group would yield a higher tissue Po_2 and develop surgical wound infections at a lower rate. Oxygen saturation, Pao_2 and tissue Po_2 were monitored during the perioperative period until 2 hours after surgery. The results revealed infection rates of 5.2% in the 80% supplemental oxygen group and 11.2% in the 30% group. Greif and colleagues concluded that perioperative supplemental oxygen administration reduced the incidence of surgical wound infections by approximately 50%.

Glucose Control

Scientific data have shown that on achieving adequate blood glucose control (GC), it is possible to overcome the deleterious effects of DM on bone and soft tissue healing.[23] By normalization of various early and late parameters of the healing process, adequate GC can potentially allow for significant improvement of clinical outcomes and patient functioning.

Several studies in various surgical subspecialties have described the effect of adequate GC on the clinical outcomes in patients with DM.[68–72] GC in diabetic cardiac surgery patients has been shown to significantly reduce deep wound infections and mortality; with those patients in whom optimal GC was achieved, the risk of infection was equal to that in nondiabetic patients.[68] Similarly, the DIGAMI study[69] related hyperglycemic patients with acute myocardial infarctions and found a significantly lower mortality rate in the group treated with insulin infusion compared with the nontreatment group. Furthermore, studies involving GC in intensive care unit (ICU) patients have also been performed.[70–72] Collectively, they reported a significant reduction in mortality, sepsis, need for dialysis, need for blood transfusions, and length of ICU stay.

The effect of GC in patients undergoing orthopedic surgery has also been evaluated. Several retrospective studies have described various complications of total joint arthroplasty in diabetic patients, namely wound complications and deep infections, urinary tract infections, and death secondary to myocardial infarction.[73–78] Some investigators have demonstrated that after total joint arthroplasty, diabetic patients are more likely than nondiabetic patients to develop these described complications.[77,78] In addition, several small retrospective studies analyzing the outcomes in patients undergoing spinal surgery have shown a significantly higher rate of infection and wound complications in diabetic patients than in nondiabetic patients.[79–81]

With reference to foot and ankle surgery, Younger and colleagues,[82] in a retrospective study, analyzed the factors affecting wound healing in 68 diabetic patients undergoing transmetatarsal amputation (TMA). Twenty-one patients with successful TMA were compared with 21 patients with failed TMA requiring further transtibial amputation (TTA), and various local and systemic factors (patient demographics, smoking, need for renal dialysis, GC, signs of peripheral vascular disease, presence of diabetic foot ulcers) were assessed for statistical relation. Younger and colleagues[81] found that glycosylated hemoglobin (HbA_{1c}), which reflects the ambient mean blood glucose level over a 2- to 3-month period, was significantly higher in the TTA group versus those patients with successful TMA. This study highlighted the importance of GC in patients with DM, as GC was shown to be the most significant factor in achieving successful clinical outcomes with regard to wound healing. However, although several clinical studies in the orthopedic literature have shown that normalizing glucose levels results in significantly reduced wound complication and infection rates and overall morbidity, the effect of GC on osseous healing has not yet been investigated in the clinical arena. Therefore, to definitively describe the effect of GC in diabetic patients undergoing foot and ankle surgery for fracture repair or elective arthrodesis, data obtained from prospective randomized clinical trials are needed.

Biophysical Stimulation

Several options are currently available for clinicians to promote the healing of fractures and accelerate the rate of union in elective arthrodesis, including the utility of biophysical stimulators, namely LIPUS (**Fig. 11**), and electrical bone stimulation devices such as pulsed electromagnetic field (PEMF) and direct current (DC). A Canadian survey of 450 trauma surgeons, with a response rate of 60%, found that 45% of surgeons reported using bone stimulators to manage tibial fractures, with their use evenly divided between LIPUS and PEMF therapy.[83] The specific literature on the use of LIPUS and PEMF in foot and ankle orthopedics is reviewed here, with a focus on patients with DM.

LIPUS

The FDA approved the use of LIPUS for acceleration of healing of conservatively managed fresh fracture healing in 1994, and for treatment of established nonunions in 2000.[84] In vitro and animal experimental studies suggest that beneficial effects of LIPUS on bone healing may include a positive impact on signal transduction, gene expression, blood flow, and tissue modeling and remodeling.[85]

Based on the clinical data, LIPUS reduces time to heal (approximately 40%) in nonoperatively managed radius and tibial fractures by a mean of 32 days (154 vs 122 days).[86] Heckman and colleagues,[87] and later Kristiansen and colleagues,[88] studied the influence of LIPUS on the healing rate of acute tibial shaft and distal radius fractures, respectively. Both showed a significant reduction in time to achieve union, and neither of the studies reported any complications from the ultrasound. Cook and colleagues[86] further evaluated the data from Heckman and showed a reduction in the number of delayed unions with the use of ultrasound bone stimulation despite smoking. One economic analysis estimated savings of $13,259 per fracture.[89] This economic analysis considered both direct and indirect costs; however, data for this model were based on a case series of 60 patients and an ultrasound registry, using radiographic healing as a surrogate for functional recovery.

Limited studies currently exist regarding the efficacy of LIPUS in fracture healing in animals with experimental diabetes. Gebauer and colleagues[90] examined the role of LIPUS in fresh femoral fracture healing in type I DM BB Wistar rats. In this study, although LIPUS did not affect the early proliferative phase of fracture healing, application of LIPUS clearly resulted in improved mechanical properties during the late phase of fracture healing, despite poor GC. Mechanical testing revealed significantly greater torque to failure and stiffness in the LIPUS-treated diabetic group compared with the non-LIPUS–treated diabetic group at 6 weeks after fracture. These findings suggest a potential role of LIPUS as an adjunct in DM fracture healing.

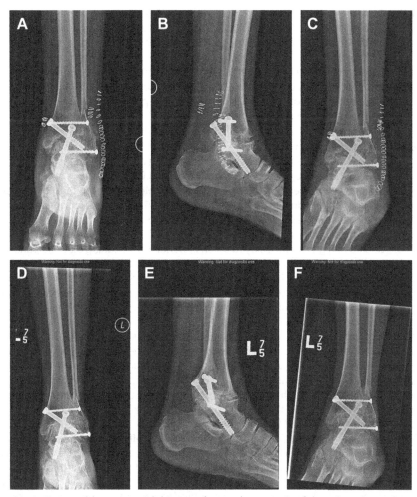

Fig. 11. A 40-year-old woman with history of avascular necrosis of the talus who underwent an ankle fusion. Postoperative radiographs at 4 months show delayed union of the attempted fusion site as seen on anteroposterior (A), lateral (B), and mortise (C) views of the ankle. Low-intensity pulsed ultrasonography was initiated at that time. Follow-up films demonstrate union at the fusion site at 6 months after intervention, as seen on anteroposterior (D), lateral (E), and mortise (F) views of the ankle.

Specific studies on the effect of LIPUS on elective fusion in patients with diabetes do not exist, but one may extrapolate from the current literature studying LIPUS on elective foot and ankle fusions. In a 12-month prospective study, Coughlin and colleagues[17] evaluated the healing rate and clinical results of patients undergoing primary subtalar arthrodeses with adjuvant LIPUS. Fifteen consecutive patients participated in the study, obtaining routine radiographs, computed tomography (CT) scans, and clinical outcomes. The clinical and radiographic data were compared with those from a similar cohort of patients, previously reported on, who had not received ultrasound bone stimulation. Results of the patients who received ultrasound bone stimulation showed a statistically significantly faster healing rate on plain radiographs at

9 weeks (*P* = .034) and CT scan at 12 weeks (*P* = .017). A 100% fusion rate was noted. The American Orthopedic Foot and Ankle Society (AOFAS) ankle and hindfoot score was also improved at 12 months postoperatively, a finding that was statistically significant (*P* = .026). The study by Coughlin and colleagues[17] is unique in being the first article to prospectively evaluate ultrasound bone stimulation in primary hindfoot arthrodesis patients. Although these patients did not have DM (actually an exclusion criterion), the faster rate of healing demonstrates the potential role of LIPUS in the high-risk elective arthrodesis patient.

Electrical bone stimulation

With respect to foot and ankle surgery in high-risk patients, 2 techniques of electrical bone stimulation have been well described: PEMF and DC.

PEMF devices use pulses of exogenous electrical potentials in the form of an electromagnetic field applied locally to the area of interest (fracture and/or nonunion site) to accelerate osseous healing. PEMF devices are worn directly on the skin or a cast, and are therefore a noninvasive method of augmenting bone healing in the management of patients at high risk for delayed union or nonunion, including diabetic patients. Long periods of use, ranging from 3 to 10 hours a day depending on the system, are recommended, whereas application for less than the recommended minimal period of 3 hours per day has been shown to significantly reduce the efficacy of electrical bone stimulation with respect to union.[91] Hence, patient noncompliance is a major potential issue.

DC devices are internally applied with a subcutaneously placed battery unit that houses the anode and an attached titanium cathode wire electrode placed into the fracture or fusion site. Although the electrical current can be delivered at maximal intensity for constant stimulation at the operative site, and patient compliance is rarely an issue, DC devices have their own disadvantages, namely local irritation or pain at the site of hardware implantation and the potential need for a secondary procedure for hardware removal in case of infection (**Fig. 12**).

Several studies[92–94] have demonstrated the beneficial effect of electrostimulation in the treatment of primary hindfoot fusions, whereas only one prospective study[94] has described the clinical application of PEMF in primary foot and ankle arthrodesis.

Dhawan and colleagues[94] performed a clinical trial consisting of 64 patients (144 joints) undergoing elective triple or subtalar arthrodesis (primary and revision) randomized into 2 groups (with and without postoperative PEMF). The study excluded patients considered to be at high risk for impaired bone healing, specifically those with rheumatoid arthritis, diabetes, or corticosteroid use. Blinded radiographic analysis was performed to assess fusion. The mean time to achieve union for the PEMF group was 12.9 weeks for primary subtalar fusions (100% unions), 12.2 weeks for talonavicular fusions, and 13.1 weeks for calcaneocuboid fusions, whereas the corresponding fusions in the non-PEMF control group demonstrated an average time to achieve union of 14.5 weeks, 17.6 weeks, and 17.7 weeks, respectively. Although determining time to union by assessing standard radiographs is not a reliable method for quantifying this end point[17] and no sham PEMF units for controls were used, this randomized prospective study showed a statistically significant reduction in time required for union in the talonavicular and calcaneocuboid fusion groups treated with PEMF and a trend toward faster union in the subtalar arthrodesis group. Of note, patients who had PEMF treatment for multiple joint arthrodeses showed a tendency for the remaining joints to fuse quicker when one of the joints fused rapidly.

Donley and Ward[93] conducted a case series to assess the outcome of DC device implantation and subsequent electrical bone stimulation in 13 patients with primary

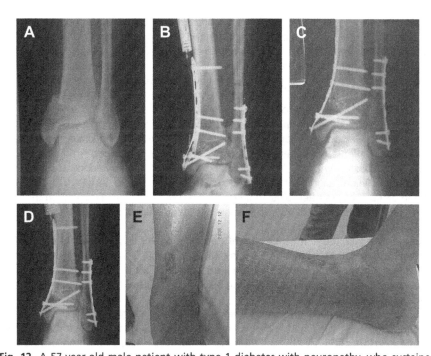

Fig. 12. A 57-year-old male patient with type 1 diabetes with neuropathy, who sustained ankle injury after falling 3 weeks before presentation in the emergency room. Preoperative anteroposterior view (*A*) of the left ankle demonstrates a distal tibia-fibula fracture. Surgical intervention consisted of ORIF of the distal tibia-fibula fracture and implantation of a DC electrical bone stimulation device (*B*). Six-week postoperative anteroposterior view of the ankle shows increasing consolidation at the fracture site (*C*), with healing evident at 4 months (*D*). However, complication associated with the use of the DC device developed at 1 year post operation, as shown in the clinical picture with exposure of wire (*E, F*).

hindfoot or ankle fusions (6 tibio-talo-calcaneal, 3 ankle, 2 subtalar, and 2 tibiocalcaneal arthrodeses). All patients enrolled in this study demonstrated at least 2 risk factors for nonunion, including a history of nonunion, smoking, and osteonecrosis of the talus. Postoperative follow-up at 1 year showed successful fusion in 12 of 13 patients (92%). Clinically, postoperative pain and modified AOFAS scores at 1 year showed significant improvement when compared with preoperative scores. The only reported complications were superficial infections requiring local wound care in 4 patients, while 8 patients reported the subcutaneous battery pack to be bothersome, 4 of whom underwent surgical removal.

Although the results of these investigations[92–94] show a positive influence of electrical bone stimulation on the fusion rates in foot and ankle primary arthrodeses, and are therefore promising, there is insufficient evidence to support the routine use of PEMF or DC devices in primary arthrodesis. In addition, the use of invasive DC devices with its concomitant risks over PEMF devices for primary arthrodesis is not supported by sufficient clinical data.

Because foot and ankle arthrodesis procedures pose a high nonunion risk, considerable interest has been generated regarding the application of electrostimulation to revision arthrodeses. However, only one case series by Saltzman and colleagues[95] has described the effect of PEMF on revision arthrodesis. In this retrospective study,

19 patients who developed nonunion after primary foot and ankle arthrodeses were treated with PEMF, immobilization, and limited weight bearing. Only 5 of the 19 patients went on to achieve union, whereas 9 of the remaining 14 underwent revision surgery, yielding similar fusion rates (2 of 9). Patients' risk factors included smoking (5 patients) and previous nonunions (8 patients). The investigators hypothesized that the lower rate of success of PEMF for revision arthrodesis of the foot and ankle, when compared with its application on long bones,[96–100] may be attributable to mechanical difficulties in orienting the coils around the foot and ankle.

Contrary to Saltzman's results, Midis and Conti[101] reported a case series of 10 consecutive patients with aseptic nonunions of the ankle requiring revision arthrodesis, supplemented with DC bone stimulation. Radiographic evidence showed that acceptable clinical alignment and solid fusion was achieved in all 10 patients at a mean of 12.8 weeks after revision surgery. In addition, clinical examination through a modified AOFAS ankle/hindfoot scoring system showed 70% good to excellent results.

In view of the limited number of clinical studies and their associated findings, which demonstrate inconsistent outcomes, it is difficult to justify the utility of electrical bone stimulation on foot and ankle revision arthrodeses. Furthermore, contrary to the previous indications, limited data exist to support the use of DC devices over PEMF devices for revision arthrodesis.

Nonunion and delayed union occur frequently in certain high-risk foot and ankle fractures, such as tibial (shaft and pilon) and metaphyseal-diaphyseal fifth metatarsal fractures. In an effort to prevent these potential complications, some orthopedic surgeons have used electrical bone stimulation on fresh fractures. However, there is no peer-reviewed literature at this time that demonstrates the beneficial effect of the utility of electrical bone stimulation on fresh fracture healing. Therefore, prospective, randomized controlled studies are required before routine clinical use can be considered in this scenario.

SUMMARY

Patients with DM undergoing foot and ankle surgery are at a greater risk for postoperative complications associated with impaired bone and soft tissue healing when compared with nondiabetic patients. With recent advances in orthopedic surgery, many options are now available to successfully manage and potentially reduce the rate of postoperative infection and wound complications, and decrease the time to achieve osseous union in this high-risk patient population. Future prospective studies investigating the use of nonconventional treatment modalities such as orthobiologics and biophysical stimulation may provide further insight as to the potential of these adjuncts to augment the diabetic healing process and improve clinical outcomes in diabetic patients after foot and ankle surgery.

REFERENCES

1. American Diabetes Association. Diabetes statistics. 2007. Available at: http://www.diabetes.org/diabetes-statistics.jsp. Accessed January 4, 2010.
2. Diabetes data and trends - CDC. Available at: http://apps.nccd.cdc.gov/DDTSTRS/default.aspx. Accessed January 4, 2010.
3. Chahal J, Stephen DJ, Bulmer B, et al. Factors associated with outcome after subtalar arthrodesis. J Orthop Trauma 2006;20(8):555–61.
4. Cozen L. Does diabetes delay fracture healing? Clin Orthop 1972;82:134–40.

5. Loder RT. The influence of diabetes mellitus on the healing of closed fractures. Clin Orthop 1988;232:210–6.
6. Papa J, Myerson M, Girard P. Salvage, with arthrodesis, in intractable diabetic neuropathic arthropathy of the foot and ankle. J Bone Joint Surg Am 1993; 75(7):1056–66.
7. Perlman MH, Thordarson DB. Ankle fusion in a high risk population: an assessment of nonunion risk factors. Foot Ankle Int 1999;20(8):491–6.
8. Stuart MJ, Morrey BF. Arthrodesis of the diabetic neuropathic ankle joint. Clin Orthop 1990;253:209–11.
9. Tisdel CL, Marcus RE, Heiple KG. Triple arthrodesis for diabetic peritalar neuroarthropathy. Foot Ankle Int 1995;16(6):332–8.
10. Einhorn TA. Enhancement of fracture-healing. J Bone Joint Surg Am 1995;77(6): 940–56.
11. Einhorn TA. The cell and molecular biology of fracture healing. Clin Orthop 1998;(355 Suppl):S7–21.
12. Einhorn TA. Clinical applications of recombinant human BMPs: early experience and future development. J Bone Joint Surg Am 2003;85(Suppl 3):82–8.
13. Hollinger JO, Hart CE, Hirsch SN, et al. Recombinant human platelet-derived growth factor: biology and clinical applications. J Bone Joint Surg Am 2008; 90(Suppl 1):48–54.
14. Lieberman JR, Daluiski A, Einhorn TA. The role of growth factors in the repair of bone. Biology and clinical applications. J Bone Joint Surg Am 2002;84(6):1032–44.
15. Chou LB, Coughlin MT, Hansen S Jr, et al. Osteoarthritis of the ankle: the role of arthroplasty. J Am Acad Orthop Surg 2008;16(5):249–59.
16. Coughlin MJ, Grimes JS, Traughber PD, et al. Comparison of radiographs and CT scans in the prospective evaluation of the fusion of hindfoot arthrodesis. Foot Ankle Int 2006;27(10):780–7.
17. Coughlin MJ, Smith BW, Traughber P. The evaluation of the healing rate of subtalar arthrodeses, part 2: the effect of low-intensity ultrasound stimulation. Foot Ankle Int 2008;29(10):970–7.
18. Kesani AK, Gandhi A, Lin SS. Electrical bone stimulation devices in foot and ankle surgery: types of devices, scientific basis, and clinical indications for their use. Foot Ankle Int 2006;27(2):148–56.
19. Kagel EM, Einhorn TA. Alterations of fracture healing in the diabetic condition. Iowa Orthop J 1996;16:147–52.
20. Praemer A, Rice D. Furner S. Frequency of occurrence. In: Praemer A, editor. Musculoskeletal conditions in United States. 1st edition. Rosemont (IL): American Academy of Orthopaedic Surgeons; 1992. p. 83–8.
21. Frey C, Halikus NM, Vu-Rose T, et al. A review of ankle arthrodesis: predisposing factors to nonunion. Foot Ankle Int 1994;15(11):581–4.
22. Coetzee JC, Pomeroy GC, Watts JD, et al. The use of autologous concentrated growth factors to promote syndesmosis fusion in the Agility total ankle replacement. A preliminary study. Foot Ankle Int 2005;26(10):840–6.
23. Beam HA, Parsons JR, Lin SS. The effects of blood glucose control upon fracture healing in the BB Wistar rat with diabetes mellitus. J Orthop Res 2002;20(6): 1210–6.
24. Funk JR, Hale JE, Carmines D, et al. Biomechanical evaluation of early fracture healing in normal and diabetic rats. J Orthop Res 2000;18(1):126–32.
25. Gooch HL, Hale JE, Fujioka H, et al. Alterations of cartilage and collagen expression during fracture healing in experimental diabetes. Connect Tissue Res 2000;41(2):81–91.

26. Macey LR, Kana SM, Jingushi S, et al. Defects of early fracture-healing in experimental diabetes. J Bone Joint Surg Am 1989;71(5):722–33.

27. Boddenberg U. [Healing time of foot and ankle fractures in patients with diabetes mellitus: literature review and report on own cases]. Zentralbl Chir 2004;129(6):453–9 [in German].

28. Donnato K. Fractures of the ankle. In: Mizel M, Miller R, Scioli M, editors. Orthopaedic knowledge update - foot & ankle 2. Rosemont (IL): American Academy of Orthopaedic Surgeons; 1998. p. 185–200.

29. Sirkin M, Sanders R, DiPasquale T, et al. A staged protocol for soft tissue management in the treatment of complex pilon fractures. J Orthop Trauma 1999;13(2):78–84.

30. Sirkin M, Sanders R, DiPasquale T, et al. A staged protocol for soft tissue management in the treatment of complex pilon fractures. J Orthop Trauma 2004;18(Suppl 8):S32–8.

31. Bibbo C, Lin SS, Beam HA, et al. Complications of ankle fractures in diabetic patients. Orthop Clin North Am 2001;32(1):113–33.

32. Sirkin M, Sanders R. The treatment of pilon fractures. Orthop Clin North Am 2001;32(1):91–102.

33. Thordarson DB. Complications after treatment of tibial pilon fractures: prevention and management strategies. J Am Acad Orthop Surg 2000;8(4):253–65.

34. Haley RW, Culver DH, Morgan WM, et al. Identifying patients at high risk of surgical wound infection. A simple multivariate index of patient susceptibility and wound contamination. Am J Epidemiol 1985;121(2):206–15.

35. Allen DB, Maguire JJ, Mahdavian M, et al. Wound hypoxia and acidosis limit neutrophil bacterial killing mechanisms. Arch Surg 1997;132(9):991–6.

36. Chang N, Goodson WH 3rd, Gottrup F, et al. Direct measurement of wound and tissue oxygen tension in postoperative patients. Ann Surg 1983;197(4):470–8.

37. Jonsson K, Jensen JA, Goodson WH 3rd, et al. Assessment of perfusion in postoperative patients using tissue oxygen measurements. Br J Surg 1987;74(4):263–7.

38. Akca O, Melischek M, Scheck T, et al. Postoperative pain and subcutaneous oxygen tension. Lancet 1999;354(9172):41–2.

39. McCormack RG, Leith JM. Ankle fractures in diabetics. Complications of surgical management. J Bone Joint Surg Br 1998;80(4):689–92.

40. Flynn JM, Rodriguez-del Rio F, Piza PA. Closed ankle fractures in the diabetic patient. Foot Ankle Int 2000;21(4):311–9.

41. White CB, Turner NS, Lee GC, et al. Open ankle fractures in patients with diabetes mellitus. Clin Orthop Relat Res 2003;414:37–44.

42. Costigan W, Thordarson DB, Debnath UK. Operative management of ankle fractures in patients with diabetes mellitus. Foot Ankle Int 2007;28(1):32–7.

43. Kline AJ, Gruen GS, Pape HC, et al. Early complications following the operative treatment of pilon fractures with and without diabetes. Foot Ankle Int 2009; 30(11):1042–7.

44. Wukich DK. Surgical site infection in foot and ankle surgery: a comparison of patients with and without diabetes mellitus. 25th Annual Summer Meeting of the American Orthopaedic Foot and Ankle Society. Vancouver, British Columbia, July 16–18, 2009.

45. Schon LC, Marks RM. The management of neuroarthropathic fracture-dislocations in the diabetic patient. Orthop Clin North Am 1995;26(2):375–92.

46. Koval KJ, Petraco DM, Kummer FJ, et al. A new technique for complex fibula fracture fixation in the elderly: a clinical and biomechanical evaluation. J Orthop Trauma 1997;11(1):28–33.

47. Dunn WR, Easley ME, Parks BG, et al. An augmented fixation method for distal fibular fractures in elderly patients: a biomechanical evaluation. Foot Ankle Int 2004;25(3):128–31.

48. Perry MD, Taranow WS, Manoli A 2nd, et al. Salvage of failed neuropathic ankle fractures: use of large-fragment fibular plating and multiple syndesmotic screws. J Surg Orthop Adv 2005;14(2):85–91.

49. Needleman RL, Skrade DA, Stiehl JB. Effect of the syndesmotic screw on ankle motion. Foot Ankle 1989;10(1):17–24.

50. Jani MM, Ricci WM, Borrelli J Jr, et al. A protocol for treatment of unstable ankle fractures using transarticular fixation in patients with diabetes mellitus and loss of protective sensibility. Foot Ankle Int 2003;24(11):838–44.

51. Gardner MJ, Brophy RH, Campbell D, et al. The mechanical behavior of locking compression plates compared with dynamic compression plates in a cadaver radius model. J Orthop Trauma 2005;19(9):597–603.

52. Liporace FA, Gupta S, Jeong GK, et al. A biomechanical comparison of a dorsal 3.5-mm T-plate and a volar fixed-angle plate in a model of dorsally unstable distal radius fractures. J Orthop Trauma 2005;19(3):187–91.

53. Alsousou J, Thompson M, Hulley P, et al. The biology of platelet-rich plasma and its application in trauma and orthopaedic surgery: a review of the literature. J Bone Joint Surg Br 2009;91(8):987–96.

54. Gandhi A, Bibbo C, Pinzur M, et al. The role of platelet-rich plasma in foot and ankle surgery. Foot Ankle Clin 2005;10(4):621–37, viii.

55. Gandhi A, O'Connor JP, Parsons JR, et al. Localized insulin delivery normalizes the impairment of the late phase of diabetic fracture healing. Paper presented at: Orthopaedic Research Society. New Orleans (LA), February 2–5, 2003.

56. Barrow CR, Pomeroy GC. Enhancement of syndesmotic fusion rates in total ankle arthroplasty with the use of autologous platelet concentrate. Foot Ankle Int 2005;26(6):458–61.

57. Saltzman CL, Alvine FG. The Agility total ankle replacement. Instr Course Lect 2002;51:129–33.

58. Pyevich MT, Saltzman CL, Callaghan JJ, et al. Total ankle arthroplasty: a unique design. Two to twelve-year follow-up. J Bone Joint Surg Am 1998;80(10): 1410–20.

59. Pinzur MS. Use of platelet-rich concentrate and bone marrow aspirate in high-risk patients with Charcot arthropathy of the foot. Foot Ankle Int 2009;30(2): 124–7.

60. Reddi AH. Bone and cartilage differentiation. Curr Opin Genet Dev 1994;4(5): 737–44.

61. Wozney J, Rosen Bone V. morphogenic proteins and their expression. In: Noda N. editor. Cellular and molecular biology of bone. San Diego (CA): Academic Press; 1993. p. 131–167.

62. Axelrad TW, Einhorn TA. Bone morphogenetic proteins in orthopaedic surgery. Cytokine Growth Factor Rev 2009;20(5–6):481–8.

63. Bibbo C, Haskell MD. Recombinant bone morphogenetic protein-2 (rhBMP-2) in high-risk foot and ankle surgery: surgical techniques and preliminary results of a prospective, intention-to-treat study. Tech Foot Ankle Surg 2007;6(2):71–9.

64. Bibbo C, Patel DV, Haskell MD. Recombinant bone morphogenetic protein-2 (rhBMP-2) in high-risk ankle and hindfoot fusions. Foot Ankle Int 2009;30(7): 597–603.

65. Babior BM. Oxygen-dependent microbial killing by phagocytes (second of two parts). N Engl J Med 1978;298(13):721–5.

66. Hopf HW, Hunt TK, West JM, et al. Wound tissue oxygen tension predicts the risk of wound infection in surgical patients. Arch Surg 1997;132(9):997–1004 [discussion: 1005].

67. Greif R, Akca O, Horn EP, et al. Supplemental perioperative oxygen to reduce the incidence of surgical-wound infection. Outcome Research Group. N Engl J Med 2000;342(3):161–7.

68. Furnary AP, Wu Y, Bookin SO. Effect of hyperglycemia and continuous intravenous insulin infusions on outcomes of cardiac surgical procedures: the Portland diabetic project. Endocr Pract 2004;10(Suppl 2):21–33.

69. Malmberg K, Ryden L, Efendic S, et al. Randomized trial of insulin-glucose infusion followed by subcutaneous insulin treatment in diabetic patients with acute myocardial infarction (DIGAMI study): effects on mortality at 1 year. J Am Coll Cardiol 1995;26(1):57–65.

70. van den Berghe G, Wouters P, Weekers F, et al. Intensive insulin therapy in the critically ill patients. N Engl J Med 2001;345(19):1359–67.

71. Krinsley JS. Association between hyperglycemia and increased hospital mortality in a heterogeneous population of critically ill patients. Mayo Clin Proc 2003;78(12):1471–8.

72. Krinsley JS. Effect of an intensive glucose management protocol on the mortality of critically ill adult patients. Mayo Clin Proc 2004;79(8):992–1000.

73. England SP, Stern SH, Insall JN, et al. Total knee arthroplasty in diabetes mellitus. Clin Orthop Relat Res 1990;260:130–4.

74. Yang K, Yeo SJ, Lee BP, et al. Total knee arthroplasty in diabetic patients: a study of 109 consecutive cases. J Arthroplasty 2001;16(1):102–6.

75. Papagelopoulos PJ, Idusuyi OB, Wallrichs SL, et al. Long term outcome and survivorship analysis of primary total knee arthroplasty in patients with diabetes mellitus. Clin Orthop Relat Res 1996;330:124–32.

76. Menon TJ, Thjellesen D, Wroblewski BM. Charnley low-friction arthroplasty in diabetic patients. J Bone Joint Surg Br 1983;65(5):580–1.

77. Jain NB, Guller U, Pietrobon R, et al. Comorbidities increase complication rates in patients having arthroplasty. Clin Orthop Relat Res 2005;435:232–8.

78. Smith DM, Oliver CH, Ryder CT, et al. Complications of Austin Moore arthroplasty. Their incidence and relationship to potential predisposing factors. J Bone Joint Surg Am 1975;57(1):31–3.

79. Simpson JM, Silveri CP, Balderston RA, et al. The results of operations on the lumbar spine in patients who have diabetes mellitus. J Bone Joint Surg Am 1993;75(12):1823–9.

80. Arinzon Z, Adunsky A, Fidelman Z, et al. Outcomes of decompression surgery for lumbar spinal stenosis in elderly diabetic patients. Eur Spine J 2004;13(1):32–7.

81. Kawaguchi Y, Matsui H, Ishihara H, et al. Surgical outcome of cervical expansive laminoplasty in patients with diabetes mellitus. Spine (Phila Pa 1976) 2000;25(5):551–5.

82. Younger AS, Awwad MA, Kalla TP, et al. Risk factors for failure of transmetatarsal amputation in diabetic patients: a cohort study. Foot Ankle Int 2009;30(12):1177–82.

83. Busse JW, Morton E, Lacchetti C, et al. Current management of tibial shaft fractures: a survey of 450 Canadian orthopedic trauma surgeons. Acta Orthop 2008;79(5):689–94.

84. Rubin C, Bolander M, Ryaby JP, et al. The use of low-intensity ultrasound to accelerate the healing of fractures. J Bone Joint Surg Am 2001;83(2):259–70.

85. Khan Y, Laurencin CT. Fracture repair with ultrasound: clinical and cell-based evaluation. J Bone Joint Surg Am 2008;90(Suppl 1):138–44.

86. Cook SD, Ryaby JP, McCabe J, et al. Acceleration of tibia and distal radius fracture healing in patients who smoke. Clin Orthop Relat Res 1997;337:198–207.

87. Heckman JD, Ryaby JP, McCabe J, et al. Acceleration of tibial fracture-healing by noninvasive, low-intensity pulsed ultrasound. J Bone Joint Surg Am 1994; 76(1):26–34.

88. Kristiansen TK, Ryaby JP, McCabe J, et al. Accelerated healing of distal radial fractures with the use of specific, low-intensity ultrasound. A multicenter, prospective, randomized, double-blind, placebo-controlled study. J Bone Joint Surg Am 1997;79(7):961–73.

89. Heckman JD, Sarasohn-Kahn J. The economics of treating tibia fractures. The cost of delayed unions. Bull Hosp Jt Dis 1997;56(1):63–72.

90. Gebauer GP, Lin SS, Beam HA, et al. Low-intensity pulsed ultrasound increases the fracture callus strength in diabetic BB Wistar rats but does not affect cellular proliferation. J Orthop Res 2002;20(3):587–92.

91. Garland DE, Moses B, Salyer W. Long-term follow-up of fracture nonunions treated with PEMFs. Contemp Orthop 1991;22(3):295–302.

92. Lau JT, Stamatis ED, Myerson MS, et al. Implantable direct-current bone stimulators in high-risk and revision foot and ankle surgery: a retrospective analysis with outcome assessment. Am J Orthop 2007;36(7):354–7.

93. Donley BG, Ward DM. Implantable electrical stimulation in high-risk hindfoot fusions. Foot Ankle Int 2002;23(1):13–8.

94. Dhawan SK, Conti SF, Towers J, et al. The effect of pulsed electromagnetic fields on hindfoot arthrodesis: a prospective study. J Foot Ankle Surg 2004;43(2):93–6.

95. Saltzman C, Lightfoot A, Amendola A. PEMF as treatment for delayed healing of foot and ankle arthrodesis. Foot Ankle Int 2004;25(11):771–3.

96. Sharrard WJ. A double-blind trial of pulsed electromagnetic fields for delayed union of tibial fractures. J Bone Joint Surg Br 1990;72(3):347–55.

97. de Haas WG, Watson J, Morrison DM. Non-invasive treatment of ununited fractures of the tibia using electrical stimulation. J Bone Joint Surg Br 1980;62(4): 465–70.

98. Bassett CA, Mitchell SN, Schink MM. Treatment of therapeutically resistant nonunions with bone grafts and pulsing electromagnetic fields. J Bone Joint Surg Am 1982;64(8):1214–20.

99. Heckman JD, Ingram AJ, Loyd RD, et al. Nonunion treatment with pulsed electromagnetic fields. Clin Orthop Relat Res 1981;161:58–66.

100. Holmes GB Jr. Treatment of delayed unions and nonunions of the proximal fifth metatarsal with pulsed electromagnetic fields. Foot Ankle Int 1994;15(10): 552–6.

101. Midis N, Conti SF. Revision ankle arthrodesis. Foot Ankle Int 2002;23(3):243–7.

Angiosomes and Wound Care in the Diabetic Foot

Mark W. Clemens, MD[a], Christopher E. Attinger, MD[b],*

KEYWORDS

• Angiosomes • Wound care • Diabetic foot • Vascular anatomy

Successful limb salvage is dependent on detailed knowledge of the vascular anatomy of the foot and ankle. The foot and ankle are composed of 6 distinct angiosomes; three-dimensional blocks of tissue fed by source arteries with functional vascular interconnections between muscle, fascia and skin. Because the foot and ankle are an end organ, their main arteries have numerous direct arterial-arterial connections that allow alternative routes of blood flow to develop if the direct route is disrupted or compromised. Understanding the boundaries of the angiosome and the vascular connections among its source arteries provides the basis for logically rather than empirically designed incisions for tissue exposure or to plan reconstructions or amputations that ultimately preserve blood flow for a surgical wound to heal.

Ian Taylor[1] first defined the angiosome principle by expanding on the work of previous anatomists[2–9] to further define the vascular anatomy of muscle and skin. He defined an angiosome as a three-dimensional anatomic unit of tissue fed by a source artery. Taylor and Minabe[10] defined at least 40 angiosomes in the body that were interconnected by either reduced caliber choke vessels or by similar caliber anastomotic arteries.[11,12] These choke vessels can be important safety conduits that allow one angiosome to eventually provide blood flow to an adjacent angiosome if the source artery of the latter is damaged. A unified network can be created so that one source artery can provide blood flow to multiple angiosomes beyond its immediate border. Occluding or interrupting one source artery surgically manipulates the system so that blood flows through the neighboring choke vessels. This is an anatomic explanation for the delay phenomenon.[13,14] Although choke vessels provide an indirect connection among angiosomes, there are also direct arterial-arterial connections that allow blood flow to immediately bypass local obstructions in the vascular tree. The 6 angiosomes of the foot and ankle originate from the 3 main source arteries: the posterior tibial artery supplies the medial

---

Drs Clemens and Attinger have no financial disclosures.

[a] Department of Plastic Surgery, Georgetown University Medical Center, 3800 Reservoir Road Northwest, Washington, DC 20007, USA

[b] Division of Wound Healing, Department of Plastic Surgery, Georgetown University Medical Center, 1st Floor Bles Building, 3800 Reservoir Road Northwest, Washington, DC 20007, USA

* Corresponding author.

E-mail address: cattinger@aol.com

Foot Ankle Clin N Am 15 (2010) 439–464
doi:10.1016/j.fcl.2010.04.003
1083-7515/10/$ – see front matter © 2010 Elsevier Inc. All rights reserved.

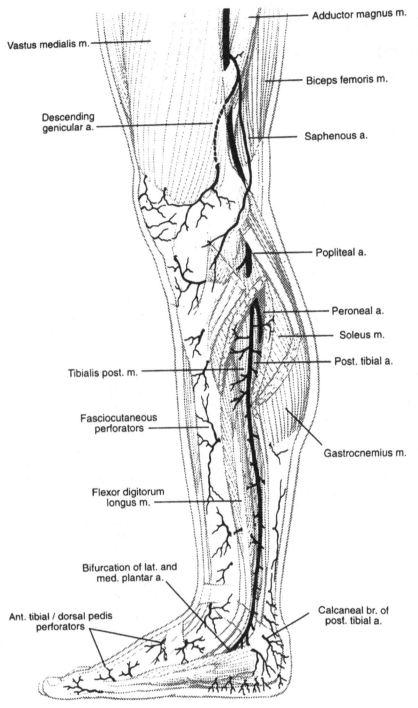

Fig. 1. The posterior tibial artery gives off perforators that arise between the flexor digitorum longus and the soleus muscle. They split into anterior and posterior branches to supply the overlying skin. (*From* Cormack GC, Lamberty BGH. The Arterial Anatomy of Skin Flaps. Edinburgh: Churchill Livingstone, 1986; with permission.)

ankle and the plantar foot, the anterior tibial artery supplies the dorsum of the foot, and the peroneal artery supplies the anterolateral ankle and the lateral rear foot. These large angiosomes of the foot can be further broken into angiosomes of the major branches of the above arteries. The 3 main branches of the posterior tibial artery each supply distinct portions of the plantar foot: the calcaneal branch (heel), the medial plantar artery (instep), and the lateral plantar artery (lateral midfoot and forefoot). The 2 branches of the peroneal artery supply the anterolateral portion of the ankle and rear foot, the anterior perforating branch (lateral anterior upper ankle), and the calcaneal branch (lateral and plantar heel). The anterior tibial artery supplies the anterior ankle and then becomes the dorsalis pedis artery, which supplies the dorsum of the foot. Detailed descriptions of the vascular anatomy[15] and angiosomes of the lower leg, foot, and ankle have been thoroughly illustrated elsewhere.[16–18]

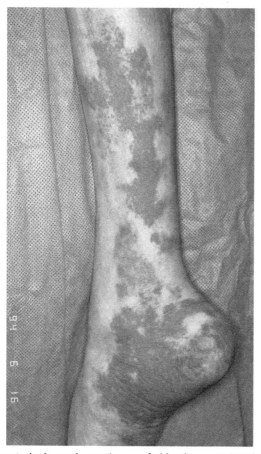

Fig. 2. This injection study shows the angiosome fed by the posterior tibial artery (*salmon*). The island of light blue just above the anterior medial malleolus comes from the peroneal artery via a direct arterial-arterial connection between the posterior tibial artery and the peroneal artery. (*Reprinted from* Attinger C. Vascular anatomy of the foot and ankle. Oper Tech Plast Reconstr Surg 1997;4:183; with permission.)

THE 3 POSTERIOR TIBIAL ARTERY ANGIOSOMES FED BY THE CALCANEAL, MEDIAL PLANTAR, AND LATERAL PLANTAR ARTERIES

In the leg, the posterior tibial artery supplies the medial lower leg, starting from the anterior medial border of the tibia and extending posteriorly to the midline of the calf over the central raphe of the Achilles tendon (**Figs. 1** and **2**). There are smaller perforator arteries along the course of the posterior tibial artery that perforate through the flexor digitorum longus and/or soleus to supply the overlying skin. In addition, there are smaller serial branches to the deep flexor muscles, the medial half of the soleus muscle, and the Achilles tendon.[16,18]

In the foot, this artery gives off the posterior medial malleolar branch at the medial malleolus. The posterior medial malleolar branch joins the anterior medial malleolar branch from the anterior tibial artery, giving rise to an important interconnection between the posterior tibial artery and the anterior tibial artery. This system supplies the medial malleolar area. At the same level, the medial calcaneal artery branches off the posterior tibial artery inferiorly and arborizes into multiple branches that travel in a coronal direction to supply the heel. The angiosome boundary of the medial calcaneal artery includes the medial and plantar heel, with its most distal boundary being the glabrous junction of the lateral posterior and plantar heel (**Figs. 3** and **4**).[19]

The posterior tibial artery then enters the calcaneal canal underneath the flexor retinaculum and bifurcates into the medial and lateral plantar arteries at the level of the transverse septum, between the abductor hallucis longus and the flexor digitorum brevis muscles. The angiosome boundaries of the medial plantar artery encompass the instep (**Fig. 5**). Its boundaries are as follows: posteriorly, the distal-medial edge of

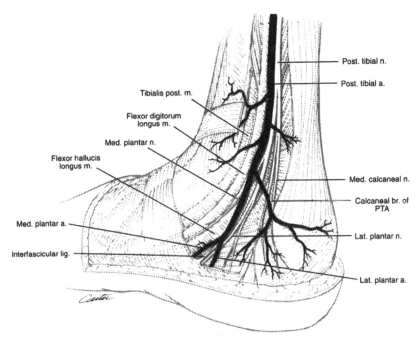

Fig. 3. The medial calcaneal branch is the first main distal branch of the posterior tibial artery. Its angiosome includes the medial heel, the plantar heel, and the lateral plantar heel up to the lateral glabrous junction. (*Reprinted from* Attinger C. Vascular anatomy of the foot and ankle. Oper Tech Plast Reconstr Surg 1997;4:183; with permission.)

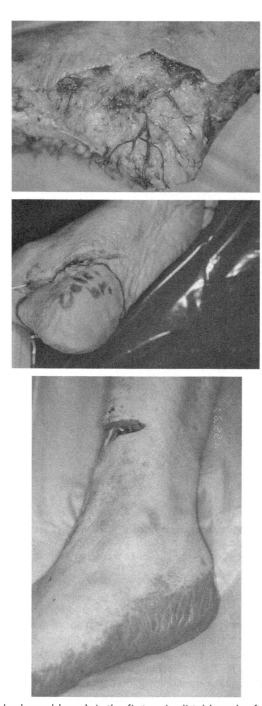

Fig. 4. The medial calcaneal branch is the first main distal branch of the posterior tibial artery (*above*). Its angiosome includes the medial heel (*center*), the plantar heel, and the lateral plantar heel up to the lateral glabrous junction (*below*). (*Reprinted from* Attinger C. Vascular anatomy of the foot and ankle. Oper Tech Plast Reconstr Surg 1997;4:183; with permission.)

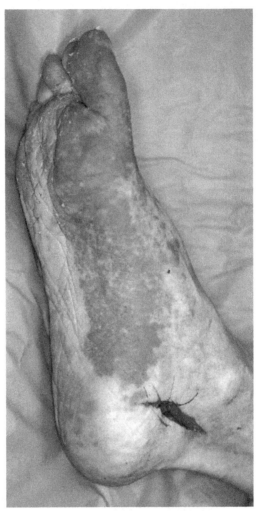

Fig. 5. The angiosome boundaries of the medial plantar artery encompass the instep and, depending on anatomic variability, can include the hallux. (*Reprinted from* Attinger C. Vascular anatomy of the foot and ankle. Oper Tech Plast Reconstr Surg 1997;4:183; with permission.)

the plantar heel; laterally, the midline of the plantar midfoot; distally, the proximal edge of the plantar forefoot; and medially, an arc 2 to 3 cm above the medial glabrous junction, with its highest point being the anterior border of the navicular-cuneiform joint.

The medial plantar artery gives off 2 main branches: the superficial and deep branches (**Figs. 6** and **7**). The superficial branch of the medial plantar artery travels obliquely up to the navicular-cuneiform joint, then along the superior border of the cuneiform and the first metatarsal bone before descending to the medial plantar aspect of the distal metatarsal. Interconnections with the anterior tibial tree exist, as cutaneous branches connect proximally with medial cutaneous branches from the dorsalis pedis artery and distally with branches of the first dorsal metatarsal artery. The artery then extends plantarly and laterally, where it joins with the deep branch

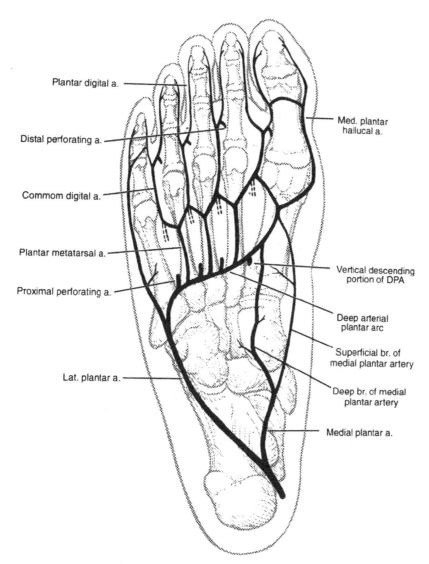

Plantar digital a.

Med. plantar
hallucal a.

Distal perforating a.

Commom digital a.

Plantar metatarsal a.

Vertical descending
portion of DPA

Proximal perforating a.

Deep arterial
plantar arc

Superficial br. of
medial plantar artery

Lat. plantar a.

Deep br. of medial
plantar artery

Medial plantar a.

Fig. 6. The medial plantar artery gives off 2 main branches: the superficial branch and the deep branch. (*Reprinted from* Attinger C. Vascular anatomy of the foot and ankle. Oper Tech Plast Reconstr Surg 1997;4:183; with permission.)

of the medial plantar artery and the first plantar metatarsal artery (a branch of the lateral plantar artery).

The second major branch of the medial plantar artery, the deep branch, travels deep and along the medial intramuscular septum between the abductor hallucis muscle and the flexor digitorum brevis. Perforating branches supply the medial sole of the foot. At the neck of the first metatarsal, it passes underneath the flexor tendons and anastomoses with the first plantar metatarsal artery and/or the distal lateral plantar artery.

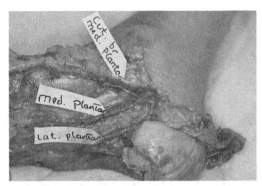

Fig. 7. The 2 main branches of the medial plantar artery are the superficial branch (cutaneous branch medial plantar) and the deep branch (medial plantar). The superficial branch travels obliquely up toward the navicular-cuneiform joint and then travels along the superior border of the cuneiform and first metatarsal bone before descending to the medial plantar aspect of the distal metatarsal. The deep branch travels along the medial intramuscular septum deep and along the fibular side of the abductor hallucis muscle. (*Reprinted from* Attinger C. Vascular anatomy of the foot and ankle. Oper Tech Plast Reconstr Surg 1997;4:183; with permission.)

The angiosome of the lateral plantar artery includes the lateral plantar surface as well as the plantar forefoot (**Fig. 8**). The borders are as follows: posteriorly, the distal lateral edge of the plantar heel; medially, the central raphe of the plantar midfoot; more distally, the glabrous juncture between the medial plantar forefoot and the medial distal dorsal forefoot; and laterally, the glabrous junction between the lateral dorsum of the foot and the plantar surface of the foot (see **Fig. 4**, below). The distal border includes the entire plantar forefoot. Although the hallux is usually part of the lateral plantar angiosome, it can also be part of the medial plantar artery angiosome (see **Fig. 5**) or of the dorsalis pedis angiosome.

The lateral plantar artery enters the middle compartment of the foot, where it travels obliquely between the flexor digitorum brevis muscle and the quadratus plantar muscle toward the base of the fifth metatarsal. It then travels distal to the proximal fifth metatarsal underneath the flexor digiti minimi muscle, turns medially, forming the deep plantar arch, and crosses the proximal (2, 3, and 4) metatarsals. It finally anastomoses directly with the dorsalis pedis artery in the proximal first interspace (**Fig. 9**). This direct anastomosis between the dorsal and plantar circulation helps ensure that if either the proximal dorsalis pedis or lateral plantar artery becomes occluded, flow is maintained to the entire foot.

The 4 plantar metatarsal arteries emanate from the deep plantar arch to nourish the plantar forefoot. They travel along each metatarsal shaft deep to the interossei and the transverse adductor muscles, but superficial to the deep transverse carpal ligament. According to Murakami,[20] they bifurcate and are joined by the deep plantar arteries and the plantar intermetatarsal arteries to form an arcade of arterial triangles. The common digital arteries arise at the apices of these triangles in the proximal web spaces. The common digital arteries bifurcate into 2 digital arteries for each toe and are joined by distal perforating branches that originate from the dorsal metatarsal arteries. The proper plantar digital arteries are the predominant blood supply to the lesser toes, except for the medial side of the second toe, which is supplied by the first metatarsal artery (see **Fig. 9**).[20]

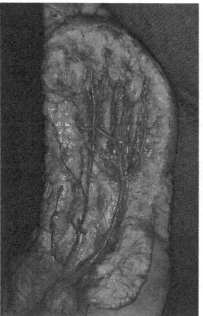 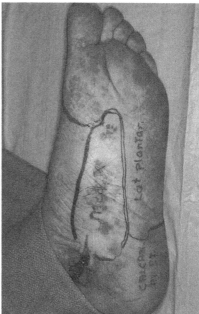

Fig. 8. The angiosome of the lateral plantar artery supplies the lateral plantar surface as well as the plantar forefoot. Its posterior border is the anterior edge of the plantar heel. Its medial border in the midfoot is the central raphe of the plantar midfoot, and in the forefoot it is the glabrous juncture between the medial dorsum and plantar forefoot. Its lateral border is the glabrous junction between the lateral dorsum of the foot and the plantar surface of the foot. The angiosome usually incorporates the hallux, although this cadaver injection shows that, occasionally, the main vascular flow of the hallux can be from the dorsal circulation. (*Reprinted from* Attinger C. Angiosomes of the foot and ankle and clinical implications for limb salvage: reconstruction, incisions, and revascularization. Plast Reconstr Surg 2006;117;261S; with permission.)

THE ANTERIOR TIBIAL ARTERY AND DORSALIS PEDIS ANGIOSOME

In the leg, the angiosome of the anterior tibial artery includes the area overlying the anterior compartment, with the fibula as the lateral boundary and the anterior tibia as the medial boundary. This artery originates from the popliteal artery and pierces the interosseus membrane to travel deep in the anterior compartment between the tibialis anterior muscle and extensor hallucis longus muscle. Proximally, it gives off muscle branches to supply the proximal third of the peroneus longus and brevis muscles. It then supplies the muscle of the anterior compartment via multiple small pedicles[10–14] to the tibialis anterior muscle, extensor hallucis longus muscle, and extensor digitorum longus muscle. At the ankle, the anterior tibial artery gives off the lateral malleolar artery at the level of the lateral malleolus that joins with the anterior perforating branch of the peroneal artery. At the same level, it also gives off the medial malleolar artery, which anastomoses with the posteromedial artery of the posterior tibial artery. The anterior tibial artery then emerges under the extensor retinaculum of the ankle to become the dorsalis pedis artery. The angiosome of the dorsalis pedis artery encompasses the entire dorsum of the foot (**Fig. 11**). This artery has arterial connections from the superficial medial plantar artery medially, from the calcaneal branch of the peroneal artery proximolaterally, and from the lateral plantar artery

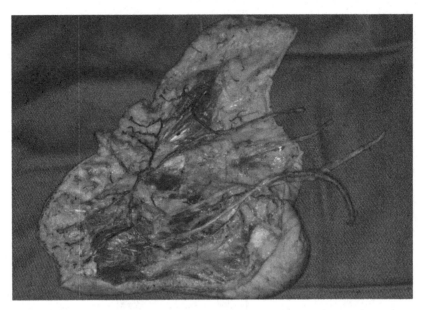

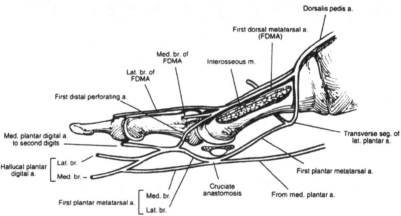

Fig. 9. (*Above*) In this cadaver specimen, all bones except for the calcaneus have been removed. Note the direct connection between the dorsalis pedis artery and the lateral calcaneal artery just distal to where Lisfranc's joint was. The two vessels create a U-shaped conduit that is critical in ensuring continued blood flow to the dorsum and plantar surfaces should the posterior tibial artery or anterior tibial artery become occluded. (*Below*) The skeletal framework shows that the dorsalis pedis artery enters into the proximal first intrametatarsal space at a 90-degree angle and then turns another 90 degrees laterally to join the lateral plantar artery. (*Reprinted from* Attinger C. Angiosomes of the foot and ankle and clinical implications for limb salvage: reconstruction, incisions, and revascularization. Plast Reconstr Surg 2006;117;261S; with permission.)

and its perforators in the proximal metatarsal interspaces. The dorsalis pedis artery travels underneath the extensor hallucis longus and curves between the extensor hallucis longus and extensor digitorum longus along the dorsum of the first interspace. As Huber[21] pointed out, the dorsalis pedis artery is absent or extremely attenuated in 12% of cases, and there are many anatomic variations to its course.

Typically, the dorsalis pedis artery has 3 lateral arterial branches (the proximal and distal tarsal arteries and the arcuate artery) and 2 medial branches (the medial tarsal arteries). The lateral branches are often linked together to form an interconnecting retelike (netlike) pattern.[22] The proximal lateral tarsal artery originates at the lateral talar neck. It travels underneath the extensor digitorum brevis muscle, giving off one or more branches to this muscle. Laterally, it communicates with the calcaneal branch of the peroneal artery. It may also connect superiorly to the lateral malleolar artery and inferiorly to the arcuate artery. The third lateral branch of the dorsalis pedis, the arcuate artery, takes off at the level of the first tarsal-metatarsal joint and travels laterally over the bases of the second, third, and fourth metatarsals. It gives off the second, third, and fourth dorsal metatarsal arteries before it joins the lateral tarsal artery. Medially, the dorsalis pedis artery (usually) gives off 2 medial tarsal arteries. One tarsal artery is located at the middle of the navicular bone, and the other is located at the cuneonavicular joint. Usually, one of these joins with the superficial branch of the medial plantar artery. After giving off the arcuate artery, the dorsalis pedis artery enters into the proximal first intermetatarsal space and in the process gives off the first dorsal metatarsal artery, which courses over the first dorsal interossei muscles. The dorsalis pedis artery enters that space by taking a 90° angle turn plantarly followed by another turn laterally to join directly with the lateral plantar artery (**Fig. 9**). In 22% of cases[23] the first dorsal metatarsal artery originates after the dorsalis pedis has made the initial downward 90° turn. In these instances, it rises toward the dorsum by traveling through the first interosseus muscle until it lies on top of the interosseus muscle at or near the metatarsophalangeal level. Regardless of its course, this artery is important because it supplies the first interosseus muscle, the skin overlying it, and the first web space. In

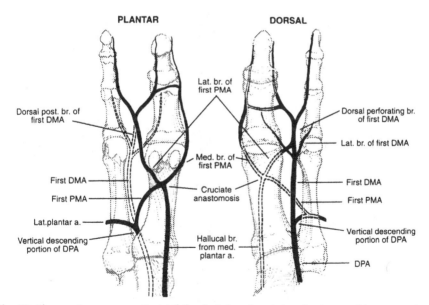

Fig. 10. The most common pattern of the first dorsal metatarsal artery and its connections with the plantar circulation is shown in dorsal and plantar views. Note the arterial-arterial connections proximally and distally in the first metatarsal interspace. (*Reprinted from* Attinger C. Vascular anatomy of the foot and ankle. Oper Tech Plast Reconstr Surg 1997;4:183; with permission.)

addition, the first dorsal metatarsal artery distally gives off medial and lateral branches that supply blood to the hallux and second digit (**Fig. 10**). The dorsal metatarsal arteries, which supply the toes, both originate from the dorsal system (the arcuate artery) and receive additional blood supply from the deep plantar system (the proximal perforating arteries) (see **Fig. 11**, left). At the metatarsal heads, the dorsal metatarsal arteries divide into 2 dorsal digital arteries and then travel to the plantar area via the distal perforating arteries (also called anterior perforating arteries). These perforating arteries join the plantar metatarsal artery to supply the plantar digits. In this way, the web space and the toes on either side of the web space receive dorsal and plantar blood supply from a dual system: the dorsalis pedis artery and the lateral plantar artery.

THE PERONEAL ARTERY FED BY THE CALCANEAL BRANCH AND ANTERIOR PERFORATING BRANCHES

The peroneal artery arises from the tibial peroneal trunk and courses along the medial side of the fibula, supplying the posterolateral lower leg, ankle, and heel.[24,25] Before the peroneal artery emerges at the level of the lateral malleolus, it bifurcates (forming a delta) into the anterior perforating branch and the lateral calcaneal branch (**Fig. 12**). The angiosome of the lateral calcaneal branch includes the plantar and lateral heel

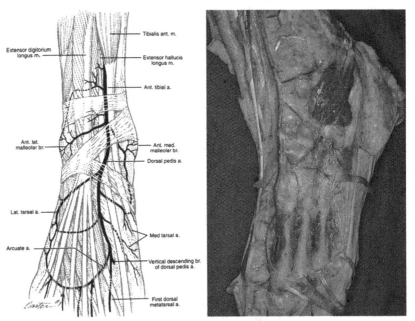

Fig. 11. The dorsalis pedis artery angiosome supplies the entire dorsum of the foot, although it gets contributions medially from the superficial medial plantar artery, anteriorly from the perforators of the lateral plantar artery, and laterally from both the calcaneal and anterior perforating branches of the peroneal artery. (*Right*) In this anatomic dissection, the arcuate artery is vestigial at best and the dorsal metatarsal arteries are getting their main blood supply from the lateral plantar artery via proximal perforators. (*From* Cormack GC, Lamberty BGH. The Arterial Anatomy of Skin Flaps. Edinburgh: Churchill Livingstone, 1986; with permission.)

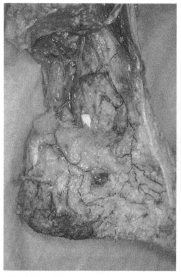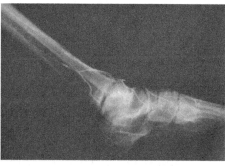

Fig. 12. Before the peroneal artery emerges at the level of the lateral malleolus, it bifurcates into the anterior perforating branch and the lateral calcaneal branch. (*Left*) The cadaver dissection shows the bifurcation after the fibula was removed. (*Right*) Angiogram view of the same bifurcation. (*Reprinted from* Attinger C. Angiosomes of the foot and clinical implications for limb salvage: reconstruction, incisions, and revascularization. Plast Reconstr Surg 2006;117:261S; with permission.)

(**Fig. 13**, left). More specifically, the proximal boundaries extend medially to the medial glabrous junction of the heel, distally to the proximal fifth metatarsal, and superiorly to the lateral malleolus. The course of the lateral calcaneal artery begins at the level of the lateral malleolus as it emerges laterally between the Achilles tendon and the peroneal tendons. It curves with peroneal tendons 2 cm distal to the lateral malleolus and gives rise to 4 or 5 small calcaneal branches.[19] The lateral calcaneal artery terminates at the level of the fifth metatarsal tuberosity, where it connects with the lateral tarsal artery. The heel is privileged in that it has 2 overlapping source arteries: the medial and lateral calcaneal arteries (**Fig. 13**, center and right). This feature ensures duplicate blood supply to an area regularly traumatized during ambulation.[26]

Anatomic and Clinical Evaluation of Arterial-arterial Connections

Arterial-arterial connections allow for uninterrupted blood flow to the entire foot despite the occlusion of one or more arteries. By understanding the location of these arterial connections in the foot and ankle, the surgeon can determine the presence of flow from the source artery and determine which artery is predominately supplying a given angiosome (**Fig. 14**). The use of the handheld Doppler instrument at the specific anatomic locations described earlier (or in any anatomic text) give an accurate description of existing blood flow.[17,27]

After locating the artery with the Doppler, the direction of flow can be evaluated by applying selective occlusion with finger pressure above and below the area being studied. The initial character of the Doppler signal helps to evaluate the quality of flow present in the artery. Triphasic flow indicates normal arterial flow. Biphasic flow indicates mildly compromised flow. Monophasic flow indicates arterial compromise, unless the patient suffers from sympathetic neuropathy (a common complication of

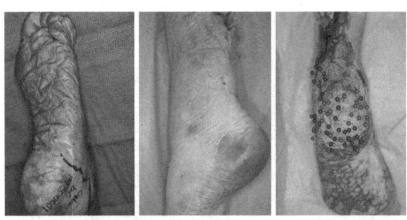

Fig. 13. The calcaneal branch of the peroneal artery supplies the entire plantar heel as well as the lateral ankle (*left*). Note that the heel is privileged in that it has 2 source arteries: the medial (*salmon*) and lateral (*blue*) calcaneal arteries. The overlap is best shown in this cadaver specimen (*center*), where each branch was injected with a different color and they completely overlap. The skin was then removed and the different colored perforators were marked with different colored pins, further emphasizing the overlap (*right*). (*Reprinted from* Attinger C. Angiosomes of the foot and ankle and clinical implications for limb salvage: reconstruction, incisions, and revascularization. Plast Reconstr Surg 2006;117; 261S; with permission.)

diabetes) and the distal vessels have lost their tone. A blunt, short, monophasic spitting sound indicates complete distal occlusion with no runoff. For example, it should be straightforward to determine whether the flow to the dorsum of the foot is derived from the anterior tibial artery, the peroneal artery (via the anterior perforating branch), or the posterior tibial artery (via the lateral plantar artery) by listening and selectively occluding these areas. In addition, one should be able to determine whether the blood flow to the heel is coming directly from the calcaneal branch of the posterior tibial artery, the calcaneal branch of the peroneal artery, or indirectly from the anterior tibial artery via the lateral malleolar branch. In the patient with diabetes mellitus and/or peripheral vascular disease who presents with a foot ulcer or rest pain, this clinical assessment can aid in choosing which incisions to make if the patient requires a debridement, amputation, or closure. In these patients it is crucial that the critically redirected blood flow is not compromised by a poorly planned surgical incision. Moreover, this directional assessment aids the vascular surgeon in ensuring that the bypass reaches the angiosome that is ischemic. It has been reported that 15% of bypasses fail to heal the foot despite remaining patent, because the bypass failed to revascularize the affected angiosome.[28]

ANTERIOR TIBIAL AND PERONEAL CONNECTIONS

The anterior tibial and peroneal arteries are directly connected through the anterior perforating branch of the peroneal artery and the lateral malleolar branch of the anterior tibial artery; thus, the flow of the peroneal artery can be retrograde from the anterior tibial artery via the lateral malleolar artery or antegrade where it supplies the anterior tibial artery (**Fig. 15**). Likewise the flow to the anterior tibial artery and the

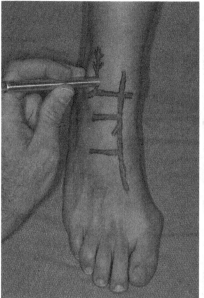 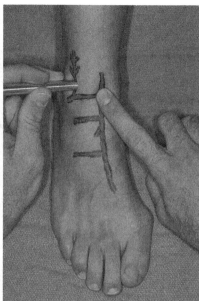

Fig. 14. The anterior perforating branch of the peroneal artery is located in the lateral soft area just above the ankle joint between the tibia and the fibula (*left*). Then, the anterior tibial artery is occluded at the takeoff of the lateral malleolar branch (*right*). If the Doppler sounds continue, then there is antegrade flow along the anterior perforating branch of the peroneal artery. (*Reprinted from* Attinger C. Angiosomes of the foot and ankle and clinical implications for limb salvage: reconstruction, incisions, and revascularization. Plast Reconstr Surg 2006;117:261S; with permission.)

dorsalis pedis can be antegrade from the proximal anterior tibial artery or retrograde from the anterior perforating branch of the peroneal artery via the lateral malleolar artery.

PERONEAL AND POSTERIOR TIBIAL CONNECTIONS

The peroneal artery communicates distally with the posterior tibial artery via 1 to 3 transverse communicating branches that are located within the fat pad deep to the Achilles tendon (**Fig. 15**). These branches are located 5 to 7 cm above the ankle joint, at the ankle joint, and just above the insertion of the Achilles tendon. Because of these connections, it is impossible by Doppler imaging to know whether the flow along the distal posterior tibial artery originates directly from the proximal posterior tibial artery or indirectly from the distal peroneal artery via the above perforators. Likewise, one cannot tell whether the flow along the peroneal artery originates from the peroneal artery or from the posterior tibial artery via those same perforators.[18]

ANTERIOR TIBIAL AND POSTERIOR TIBIAL CONNECTIONS

The anterior tibial artery and posterior tibial artery are also directly connected distal to the Lisfranc joint, where the dorsalis pedis artery enters into the proximal first

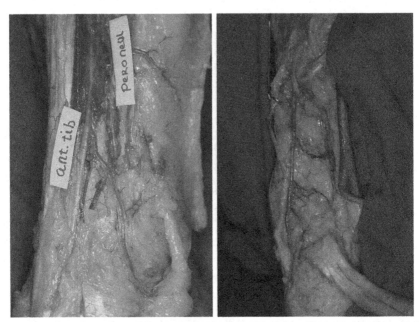

Fig. 15. The peroneal artery communicates distally with the anterior tibial artery via the anterior perforating branch and lateral malleolar artery (*left*). It also communicates distally directly with the posterior tibial artery via 1 to 3 connecting branches under the Achilles tendon (*right*). (*Reprinted from* Attinger C. Angiosomes of the foot and clinical implications for limb salvage: reconstruction, incisions, and revascularization. Plast Reconstr Surg 2006;117;261S; with permission.)

interspace to join directly with the lateral plantar artery (see **Fig. 9**). As we have previously shown,[18] the importance of evaluating the patency of the distal connection between the anterior and posterior tibial arteries cannot be emphasized enough. If that connection is critical to supplying either the dorsal or plantar surface of the foot because of existing obstruction of one of the 2 arteries, damaging that connection while performing an operation or amputation can lead to gangrene on the portion of the foot that was dependent on retrograde flow (**Fig. 16**).

ARTERIAL-ARTERIAL CONNECTIONS AROUND THE HEEL

The heel is unique in that it is the only angiosome that receives inflow from 2 source arteries: the calcaneal branch of the posterior tibial artery and the calcaneal branch of the peroneal artery (see **Fig. 13**, right). The posterior tibial calcaneal branch supplies the medial aspect of the heel, whereas the peroneal calcaneal branch supplies the lateral aspect of the heel. The former runs directly toward the heel pad along the center of the medial heel, whereas the latter curves around the lateral malleolus 2 cm distal to the malleolar tip and travels to the proximal fifth metatarsal head. There are no anatomic arterial-arterial connections between these arteries; therefore, a Doppler signal obtained in this location represents only antegrade flow. However, it is important to assess the flow in the calcaneal branch of the posterior tibial artery and the peroneal artery, to determine whether one artery predominates over the other. This

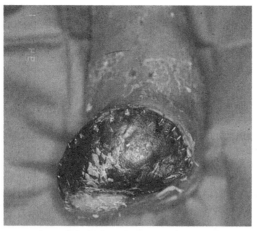

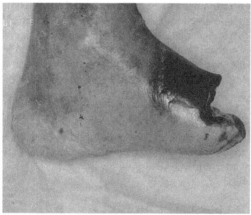

Fig. 16. (*Above*) This foot's plantar blood supply came from the dorsalis pedis artery via retrograde flow. When the amputation was performed and that connection was cut, the distal plantar surface went on to necrose. (*Below*) This foot's dorsal blood supply came from the lateral plantar artery via retrograde flow. When the amputation was performed and that connection was cut, the distal dorsal surface went on to necrose. (*Reprinted from* Attinger C. Vascular anatomy of the foot and ankle. Oper Tech Plast Reconstr Surg 1997;4:183; with permission.)

issue becomes relevant when one is planning to perform a midline Gaenslen[29] incision to expose the plantar calcaneus.

ARTERIAL-ARTERIAL CONNECTIONS OF THE PLANTAR FOOT

There are multiple levels of arterial-arterial interconnections in the plantar foot. Proximally and medially, there are the connections between the branches of the medial tarsal artery and the superficial medial plantar artery, but the medial tarsal artery is often too small to accurately examine using the Doppler device. At the Lisfranc joint, the dorsal circulation and plantar circulation are linked together via proximal perforators. Medially, the dorsalis pedis links directly with the lateral plantar artery (see **Fig. 9**).

More laterally, the dorsal and plantar metatarsal arteries are linked at their takeoff by the proximal perforating branches. At the web spaces, distal perforating arteries again link the dorsal and plantar metatarsal arteries. The final arterial-arterial interconnection is a fine subdermal arteriolar plexus linking the dorsalis pedis with the lateral plantar artery in a circumferential wraparound pattern about the plantar foot.

DORSALIS PEDIS, LATERAL PLANTAR ARTERIES, AND CRUCIATE ANASTOMOSIS

In the plantar foot, the principle connection to evaluate is that between the dorsalis pedis and lateral plantar arteries. First, use the Doppler device to examine the lateral plantar artery proximal to the base of the proximal first interspace. Then, occlude the dorsalis pedis at the tarsal-metatarsal joint. If the signal disappears, then flow in the lateral plantar artery depends on the dorsalis pedis arterial flow. However, if the sound remains, it means that there is antegrade flow from the posterior tibialis artery to the lateral plantar artery.

A second source of arterial-arterial anastomosis occurs proximal to the first metatarsal head at the cruciate anastomosis, where the superficial and deep medial plantar arteries join (see **Fig. 10**). The distal lateral plantar artery also joins the cruciate anastomosis, linking the medial plantar artery with the lateral plantar artery. The blood supply to the first toe depends on which arteries anastomose and which provide the major blood supply to the cruciate anastomosis: the medial plantar artery, lateral plantar artery, or first dorsal metatarsal artery.

The final arterial-arterial interconnection was first described by Hidalgo and Shaw,[30] who showed a fine subdermal arteriolar plexus linking the dorsalis pedis with the lateral plantar artery in a circumferential wraparound pattern about the plantar foot. They span the angiosome boundaries of the dorsalis pedis artery, medial plantar artery, and lateral plantar artery.

CONNECTIONS ON THE DORSUM OF THE FOOT

As discussed earlier, the dorsal and plantar arterial systems are closely linked at multiple levels. The most proximal is located in the medial foot, where the medial tarsal artery communicates with the superficial (medial branch) of the medial plantar artery. It is usually too difficult to use Doppler imaging on this small connection. Laterally, there is the rete that connects the proximal lateral tarsal artery, the distal tarsal and arcuate arteries, and the lateral malleolar artery and the anterior perforating branch of the peroneal superiorly. In addition, the calcaneal branch of the peroneal artery connects with the lateral tarsal artery. Because of this complex network of connections, it is difficult to determine the source of retrograde flow over the major tarsal artery when it is occluded proximally. If there is retrograde flow along the proximal lateral tarsal artery, it signifies an intact network of connections that can include the anterior perforating branch of the lateral plantar artery, the lateral malleolar artery, the calcaneal branch of the peroneal artery, the distal tarsal artery arcuate artery, and the arcuate artery. The arterial connection described in detail earlier occurs just distal to the Lisfranc joint, where the dorsalis pedis artery joins the lateral plantar artery in the proximal first interspace (see **Fig. 9**). At the proximal metatarsal interspaces and at distal web spaces, the proximal and distal perforating arteries, respectively, link the dorsal and plantar metatarsal arteries (see **Fig. 11**, left). The direction(s) of flow along the dorsal metatarsals can be easily determined. This close linkage ensures that collateral flow compensates for occlusions to either the dorsalis pedis or posterior tibial artery.

Using the Principles of Angiosomes to Make Safe Incisions in Normal and Vascularly Compromised Patients

As we have previously reported in more detail,[18] there are 4 important factors to be considered and balanced when choosing where to place an incision. The incision must provide adequate exposure for the planned procedure. In addition, there must be adequate blood supply on either side of the incision to optimize healing. Third, the incision should spare the sensory and motor nerves. Fourth, the incision should not be placed perpendicular to a joint, because of the risk of causing scar contracture and resultant joint immobility. Although adequate exposure, nerve location, and scar contracture are important factors, we focus primarily on the vascular ramifications of typical incisions in the foot and ankle.

We have described earlier in detail the importance of assessing the blood flow to each angiosome. As we stated, the presence of a palpable pulse or a Doppler-detectable triphasic sound over the source artery to a given angiosome indicates adequate blood flow to that angiosome. If there is good blood flow from the source artery feeding each angiosome, the safest incisions to make are along the border between 2 adjacent angiosomes, because each side of the incision has maximal blood flow. Therefore, incisions along the central raphe over the Achilles tendon, along the glabrous junction separating the sole of the foot from the dorsum of the foot, or along the midline of the sole of the foot are safe incisions.

One cannot reach all areas of the foot through these incisions, and blood flow to each angiosome is not always satisfactory; thus, well-deliberated compromises need to be made. When the signal of a source artery to one of 2 adjacent angiosomes is absent, the affected ischemic angiosome depends on the surrounding angiosomes for blood flow via the choke vessels. Because the choke vessels can require 4 to 10 days to become patent after a given angiosome becomes ischemic, incisions placed too soon after an arterial occlusion for collateral circulation to develop run the risk of poor healing, necrosis, or gangrene.[13,14] However, in patients with chronic arteriosclerosis, the occlusion is gradual and the choke vessels are usually patent by the time the source vessel closes.

In the vascularly compromised patient, collateral flow may keep the ischemic angiosome vascularized, and incisions must be planned so that this collateral flow is not disturbed. In the more extreme ischemic cases, in which there are no palpable pulses and the Doppler sounds are monophasic, then possible surgical revascularization should be entertained before proceeding. When one of the pulses is not present, it is best to place the incision away from the patent source artery, as we have previously reported.[18] This is the safest location, because there is minimal risk of damaging the patent source artery or the crucial choke vessels. We briefly discuss the most frequently used incisions and refer the reader to the article by Attinger and colleagues[18] for a more detailed discussion.

INCISIONS AT THE ACHILLES TENDON

Incisions over the Achilles tendon are the safest if they are made along the midline that divides the peroneal angiosome from the posterior tibial angiosome. Incisions on either side of the Achilles tendon to expose the distal tibia or fibula are also safe, provided that the posterior tibial artery and the peroneal artery are patent. The rich interconnecting vascular plexus around the Achilles tendon keeps the skin above the Achilles tendon viable. A medial to lateral S-shaped incision minimizes injury to the sural nerve and lesser saphenous vein. If an incision is made along the glabrous junction of the posterior heel, the medial portion of the incision should not extend to the medial edge of the Achilles tendon, to avoid damaging the medial calcaneal neurovascular structures. It is safer to make the incision laterally along the glabrous junction, which represents the distal angiosome boundary of the calcaneal branch of the posterior tibial artery.

INCISIONS AT THE LATERAL CALCANEUS

To expose the lateral calcaneus to treat calcaneal fractures, an L-shaped incision should be used, as advocated by Benirschke and Sangeorzan.[31] It is the safest incision if the lower portion of the incision is made along the glabrous junction between the plantar heel and the lateral heel (see **Fig. 17**, above).[19] Because the lateral heel glabrous juncture is the lateral border of the angiosome fed below by the calcaneal branch of the posterior tibial artery and above by the calcaneal branch of the peroneal artery, an incision above that glabrous juncture leaves the intervening tissue between the glabrous junction and the incision in jeopardy (see **Fig. 17**, below). In the usual trauma patient with a calcaneal fracture, the choke vessels between the posterior tibial

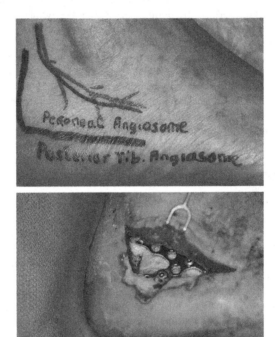

Fig. 17. The L-shaped incision, advocated by Benirschke and Sangeorzan, to expose the lateral calcaneus in calcaneus fractures should be designed with the lower portion of the incision along the glabrous junction between the plantar heel and the lateral heel (*above*). The lateral heel glabrous juncture is the boundary that represents the lateral extent of the angiosome fed by the calcaneal branch of the posterior tibial artery. An incision above the glabrous juncture into the lateral heel proper leaves the tissue between the glabrous junction and the incision in jeopardy, because that tissue lies in the just-divided angiosome of the calcaneal branch of the peroneal artery (*below*). (*Reprinted from* Attinger C. Angiosomes of the foot and ankle and clinical implications for limb salvage: reconstruction, incisions, and revascularization. Plast Reconstr Surg 2006;117:261S; with permission.)

calcaneal and peroneal calcaneal angiosomes have not had the time to open up and allow the calcaneal branch of the posterior tibial artery to feed the tissue beyond its boundary. As we stated earlier, it usually takes 4 to 10 days for the choke vessels to become patent, and it may take even longer in the setting of overlying soft-tissue damage and inflammation.[13]

INCISIONS OVER THE PLANTAR HEEL

In general, incisions over the plantar heel are reserved for hindfoot limb salvage in the presence of osteomyelitis. Safe incisions over the plantar heel from a vascular perspective can be coronal or sagittal in orientation, if the posterior tibial and peroneal arteries are patent. Whether the resultant scar is acceptable is another question.[31] Recall that the blood flow to the heel lies primarily in a coronal direction from the calcaneal branch of the posterior tibial artery (medial) and the peroneal artery (lateral). The coronal incision does not disturb the coronal flow or the sensory nerves that travel in the same direction.

If the incision is in the sagittal direction, then the flow comes to each side of the incision from the respective calcaneal arteries. However, the sensory nerves will be damaged, which is less problematic if the patient is neuropathic. In that instance, a Gaenslen[29] incision down the central heel pad is the ideal choice to expose the calcaneus for calcanectomy. Taking care to adequately evert the edges when closing the incision avoids an inverted and chronically calloused scar.

INCISIONS AT THE PLANTAR MEDIAL MIDFOOT

The plantar tissue is fed by perforators principally on either side of the plantar fascia (**Fig. 18**). If both plantar arteries open, the safest incision is along the plantar midline separating the medial plantar angiosome from the lateral plantar angiosome (**Fig. 19**, left). One can also use a curved or Z-shaped incision with the top 2 limbs following more or less along the boundary of the medial plantar artery (see **Fig. 19**, center). If a curved incision is chosen, it should have its apex laterally based to better follow the angiosome boundary between the medial and lateral plantar arteries (see **Fig. 19**, right). Care has to be taken to preserve the perforators along either side of the plantar fascia. Coronal incisions are also equally secure if the proximal and distal perforators or the underlying neurovascular bundles are not damaged.

INCISIONS ALONG THE MEDIAL AND LATERAL FOOT

For approaches to the medial midfoot, the incision is made along the border between the medial plantar artery angiosome and the dorsalis pedis angiosome (see **Fig. 5**). Two to 3 cm above the medial glabrous junction is safe, provided that the superficial and deep medial plantar arteries are open. To accurately map out the border, one should use the Doppler device to determine the course of the superficial medial plantar artery and design the incision dorsal to its course. The plantar side of the incision is then carefully lifted off the underlying bone, with care taken not to damage the superficial medial plantar artery. Alternatively, the incision can be made at the glabrous junction in the center of the medial plantar angiosome. Because 2 medial plantar arteries provide blood supply to the medial plantar angiosome, it is safe to make an incision in between them, provided they are both patent. Laterally, the safest incision is along the glabrous junction at the border between the dorsal and plantar tissue (see **Fig. 4**, below). The incision lies at the border between the dorsal foot angiosome (dorsalis pedis artery) and the plantar angiosome (lateral plantar artery).

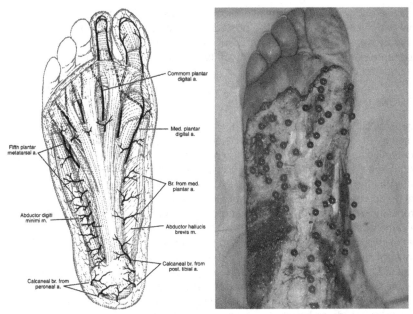

Fig. 18. Most of the perforators that feed the plantar midfoot arise along each side of the plantar fascia from the lateral plantar artery and deep medial plantar artery (*left*). The different colored pins show the location of the perforators on either side of the plantar fascia (*right*). (*Reprinted from* Attinger C. Vascular anatomy of the foot and ankle. Oper Tech Plast Reconstr Surg 1997;4:183; with permission.)

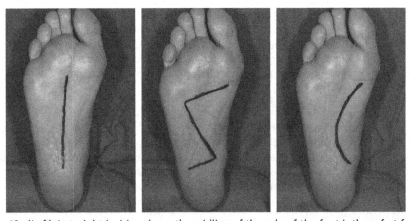

Fig. 19. (*Left*) A straight incision down the midline of the sole of the foot is the safest from a vascular perspective. (*Center*) One can also use a curved or Z-shaped incision with the top 2 limbs following more or less along the boundary of the medial plantar artery. (*Right*) If a curved incision is chosen, it should have its apex laterally based, so as to better follow the angiosome boundary between the medial and lateral plantar arteries. (*Reprinted from* Attinger C. Angiosomes of the foot and ankle and clinical implications for limb salvage: reconstruction, incisions, and revascularization. Plast Reconstr Surg 2006;117: 261S; with permission.)

INCISIONS ON THE DORSUM OF THE FOOT

When considering dorsal foot incisions, recall that the dorsal circulation proximal to the Lisfranc joint travels in a coronal direction, and distal to the Lisfranc joint it travels in a sagittal direction (see **Fig. 11**, left). The lateral proximal dorsum of the foot is composed of a rete of coronally interconnected arteries of the lateral malleolar, tarsal (proximal and distal), and arcuate arteries. This rete is linked superiorly to the anterior perforating branch and laterally to the calcaneal branch of the peroneal arteries. Medial to the dorsalis pedis artery is the medial tarsal artery, which may be directly linked to the superficial medial plantar artery. We placing the incision parallel to the direction of the arterial supply. Coronal incisions in the lateral proximal dorsal foot are parallel to the coronally directed arteries (proximal tarsal, distal tarsal, arcuate arteries, and their perforators). In addition, the dorsalis pedis artery should be identified and spared, unless it is clear that the antegrade and retrograde flow is strong. For approaches to the medial proximal dorsal foot, the safest incision is along the border between the medial plantar artery angiosome and the dorsalis pedis angiosome. For incisions of the distal forefoot, it is important not to place an incision through the metatarsal arteries, unless they both have antegrade flow (from the arcuate artery and proximal perforators) and retrograde flow (from the distal perforators). Recall that the metatarsal arteries arise from the arcuate artery, travel along the interosseus space, and are connected to plantar circulation proximally and distally by perforators. If the metatarsal artery flow is bidirectional, then coronally directed incisions are safe. However, if the flow is unidirectional, the incisions should be in the sagittal direction, over the metatarsal bones themselves, in order not to disturb the dorsal metatarsal arteries. Multiple parallel sagittal incisions over the distal dorsal forefoot can be performed as long as the dorsal metatarsal arteries are preserved. Only 3 incisions are necessary to gain access to all metatarsals, and the incisions should be short, with little undermining of the skin overlying the interosseus muscles.

INCISIONS FOR AMPUTATIONS

In general, performing forefoot and midfoot amputations in patients who have intact circulation with the dorsal and plantar antegrade blood flow has minimal risk. All incisions should be designed at the angiosome boundaries to maximize blood flow at the edges of the amputation. Medial and lateral incisions should be at the glabrous juncture between the dorsal and plantar circulation, whereas dorsal and plantar incisions should be to bone, without undermining to preserve the metatarsal arteries in the flaps. When there is compromised flow and a forefoot or midfoot amputation is planned, it is important that the remaining blood flow and arterial-arterial connections are mapped completely. If the dorsal circulation depends on the plantar circulation or vice versa, then connections between the 2 regions cannot be disturbed (see **Fig. 17**). That is, the connection between the dorsalis pedis and lateral plantar arteries at the proximal first interspace must be maintained. To preserve that connection when performing a short transmetatarsal or Lisfranc amputation, the lateral 4 metatarsals are removed laterally whereas the first metatarsal is removed medially.

Using the Angiosome Principle in Planning the Optimal Revascularization

Despite the current advances in revascularization techniques, vascular bypass surgery fails to heal approximately 15% of ischemic lower extremity wounds with a patent bypass.[28–43] Gooden and colleagues[44] found that up to 25% of patients with heel ulcers ultimately succumbed to a proximal leg amputation despite a palpable pedal pulse. The failures may be due in part to inadequate postoperative wound care,[45] but the major part of the problem is caused by the inadequate revascularization of the local ischemic area, because the vascular connections between the revascularized vessel and the source vessel nourishing the ischemic area are absent or occluded.

Thus, successful revascularization for ischemic wounds is more complex than simply restoring circulation to a specific artery. The failure of limb salvage in a percentage of successful bypasses suggests that more effective revascularization may occur if the bypassed vessel directly feeds the source artery of the angiosome containing the ulceration. That is, revascularization of the major artery directly supplying the ischemic and ulcerated angiosome should be more successful than revascularizing one of the other 2 major arteries and hoping that existing arterial-arterial connections for the blood flow reach the ischemic ulcerated angiosome.[46]

We retrospectively examined the results of direct versus indirect consecutive revascularization of 52 limbs. There was a 9.1% failure rate when wounds were directly revascularized versus a 38.1% failure rate in the wounds indirectly bypassed ($P = .03$). Those who failed to heal went on to a major leg amputation. The amputation rate, therefore, in the indirectly bypassed group was 4 times that of the directly bypassed group. This study supports the suggestion that direct revascularization of the affected angiosome leads to higher limb salvage rates.

If the vascular surgeon has more than one vessel to bypass to, or has the choice of endovascularly opening more than one vessel, they should preferentially open the vessel that directly feeds the affected angiosome. For heel wounds, the peroneal or posterior tibial artery should be preferentially revascularized. For plantar foot wounds, the posterior tibial artery should be preferentially revascularized. For lateral ankle wounds, the peroneal artery should be preferentially revascularized. For dorsal foot wounds, the anterior tibial artery should be preferentially revascularized. If the vascular surgeon cannot revascularize the source artery to the affected angiosome, they can then predict a failure rate of the revascularization to be 15% or higher unless the surgeon can show that the arterial-arterial connections between the artery to be revascularized and the source artery of the affected angiosome are open.

SUMMARY

Three major arteries supply the foot and ankle and create vascular redundancy through multiple arterial-arterial connections. A Doppler device may be used to map out the patient's vascular tree, including the direction of flow. Knowledge of the 6 angiosomes of the foot and ankle combined with an adequate Doppler examination can optimize the success of any planned treatment or procedure. This information is essential for successful limb salvage in diabetic patients and patients with peripheral vascular disease and ultimately helps a surgeon to decide whether a reconstruction is possible or an amputation is indicated.

REFERENCES

1. Taylor GI, Palmer JH. The vascular territories (angiosomes) of the body: experimental studies and clinical applications. Br J Plast Surg 1990;43:1.
2. Morain WD, Ristic J. Manchot: the cutaneous arteries of the human body. New York: Springer Verlag; 1983.
3. Salmon M. In: Taylor GI, Tempest MN, editors. Arteries of the skin. Edinburgh (UK): Churchill Livingston; 1988.
4. McGregor IA, Morgan G. Axial and random pattern flaps. Br J Plast Surg 1973; 26:202.

5. Daniel RK, Cunningham DM, Taylor GI. The deltopectoral flap: an anatomical and hemodynamic approach. Plast Reconstr Surg 1975;55:275.
6. Mathes SJ, Nahai F. Clinical atlas of muscle and musculocutaneous flaps. St Louis (MO): Mosby; 1979.
7. Ger R. Operative treatment of the advanced stasis ulcer using muscle transposition. Am J Surg 1970;120:376.
8. Orticochea M. The musculocutaneous flap method: an immediate and heroic substitute for the method of delay. Br J Plast Surg 1972;25:106.
9. McCraw JB, Dibell DG. Experimental definition of independent myocutaneous vascular territories. Plast Reconstr Surg 1977;60:341.
10. Taylor GI, Minabe T. The angiosomes of the mammals and other vertebrates. Plast Reconstr Surg 1992;89:181.
11. Calligari PR, Taylor GI, Caddy CM, et al. An anatomic review of the delay phenomenon: I. Experimental studies. Plast Reconstr Surg 1992;89:397.
12. Taylor GI, Corlett RJ, Caddy CM, et al. An anatomic review of the delay phenomenon: II. Clinical applications. Plast Reconstr Surg 1992;89:408.
13. Morris SF, Taylor GI. The time sequence of the delay phenomenon: when is a surgical delay effective? An experimental study. Plast Reconstr Surg 1995;95:526.
14. Dhar SC, Taylor GI. The delay phenomenon: the story unfolds. Plast Reconstr Surg 1999;104:2079.
15. Sarrafian SK. Anatomy of the foot and ankle. Philadelphia: Lippincott; 1993. pp. 294–355.
16. Taylor GI, Pan WR. Angiosomes of the leg: anatomic study and clinical implications. Plast Reconstr Surg 1998;102:599.
17. Attinger CE, Evans KK, Bulan E, et al. Angiosomes of the foot and ankle clinical implications for limb salvage: reconstruction, incisions, and revascularization. Plast Reconstr Surg 2006;117:261S–93S.
18. Attinger CE, Cooper P, Blume P, et al. The safest surgical incision and amputations applying the angiosomes principle and using the Doppler to assess the arterial-arterial connections of the foot and ankle. Foot Ankle Clin North Am 2001;6:745.
19. Attinger C, Cooper P. Soft tissue reconstruction for calcaneal fractures or osteomyelitis. Orthop Clin North Am 2001;32:135.
20. Murakami T. On the position and course of the deep plantar arteries, with special reference to the so called plantar metatarsal arteries. Okajimas Folia Anat Jpn 1971;48:295.
21. Huber JF. The arterial network supplying the dorsum of the foot. Anat Rec 1941;80:373.
22. Adachi B. Das arteriensystem der Japaner. Kyoto (Japan): Maruzen; 1928. pp. 246–48.
23. May JW, Chait LA, Cohen BE. Free neurovascular flap from the first web of the foot in hand reconstruction. J Hand Surg Am 1977;5:387.
24. Shusterman MA, Reece GP, Milller MJ. The osteocutaneous free fibula flap: is the skin paddle reliable? Plast Reconstr Surg 1992;90:787.
25. Jones NF, Monstrey MD, Gambier BA. Reliability of the fibular osteocutaneous flap for mandibular reconstruction: anatomical and surgical confirmation. Plast Reconstr Surg 1996;97:707.
26. Masqualet AC, Beveridge J, Romana C. The lateral supramalleolar flap. Plast Reconstr Surg 1988;81:74.
27. Taylor GI, Doyle M, McCarten G. The Doppler probe for planning flaps: anatomical study and clinical applications. Br J Plast Surg 1990;43:1.

28. Berceli SA, Chan AK, Pomposelli FB, et al. Efficacy of dorsal pedal artery bypass in limb salvage for ischemic heel ulcers. J Vasc Surg 1999;30:499.

29. Gaenslen FJ. Split heel approach in osteomyelitis of the os calcis. J Bone Joint Surg 1931;13:759.

30. Hidalgo DA, Shaw WW. Anatomic basis of plantar flap design. Plast Reconstr Surg 1986;78:267.

31. Benirschke SK, Sangeorzan BJ. Extensive intra-articular fractures of the foot: surgical management of calcaneal fractures. Clin Orthop 1993;291:128.

32. Jahss MH. Surgical principles and the plantigrade foot. In: Jahss MH, editor. Disorder of the foot and ankle: medical and surgical management. 2nd edition. Philadelphia: Saunders; 1991. p. 236–79.

33. Treiman GS, Oderich GS, Ashrafi A, et al. Management of ischemic heel ulceration and gangrene: an evaluation of factors associated with successful healing. J Vasc Surg 2000;31:1110.

34. Carsten CG III, Taylor SM, Langan EM III, et al. Factors associated with limb loss despite a patent infrainguinal bypass graft. Am Surg 1998;64:33.

35. Edwards JM, Taylor LM, Porter JM. Limb salvage in end-stage renal disease (ESRD), comparison of modern results in patients with and without ESRD. Arch Surg 1998;123:1164.

36. Chang BB, Paty PK, Shah DM, et al. Results of infrainguinal bypass for limb salvage in patients with end-stage renal disease. Surgery 1990;108:742.

37. Andros G, Harris RW, Dulawa LB, et al. The need for arteriography in diabetic patients with gangrene and palpable foot pulses. Arch Surg 1984;119:1260.

38. Johnson BL, Glickman MH, Bandyk DF, et al. Failure of foot salvage in patients with end-stage renal disease after surgical revascularization. J Vasc Surg 1995;22:280.

39. Elliot BM, Robison JG, Brothers TE, et al. Limitations of peroneal artery bypass grafting for limb salvage. J Vasc Surg 1993;18:881.

40. Bergamini TM, George SM, Massey H, et al. Pedal or peroneal bypass: which is better when both are patent? J Vasc Surg 1994;20:347.

41. Seeger JM, Pretus HA, Carlton L, et al. Potential predictors of outcome in patients with tissue loss who undergo infrainguinal vein bypass grafting. J Vasc Surg 1999;30:427.

42. Darling RC III, Chang BB, Paty PS, et al. Choice of peroneal or dorsalis pedis artery bypass for limb salvage. Am J Surg 1995;170:109.

43. Abou-Zamzam AM, Moneta GL, Lee R, et al. Peroneal bypass is equivalent to inframalleolar bypass for ischemic pedal gangrene. Arch Surg 1996;131:894.

44. Gooden MA, Gentile AT, Mills JL, et al. Free tissue transfer to extend the limits of limb salvage for lower extremity tissue loss. Am J Surg 1997;174:644.

45. Attinger CE, Ducic I, Neville RF, et al. The relative roles of aggressive wound care versus revascularization in salvage of the threatened lower extremity in the renal failure diabetic patient. Plast Reconstr Surg 2002;109:1281.

46. Neville RF, Attinger CE, Bulan EJ, et al. Revascularization of a specific angiosome for limb salvage: Does the target artery matter? Ann of Vasc Surg 2009;23(3): 367–73.

Surgery for Diabetic Foot Infections

Daniel J. Cuttica, DO, Terrence M. Philbin, DO

KEYWORDS

• Diabetes • Foot and ankle infection • Osteomyelitis

Diabetes mellitus is a common medical problem in the world today. According to the American Diabetes Association, there are 23.6 million people in the United States suffering from diabetes mellitus, which is approximately 8% of the population. Of those, 24% of cases are undiagnosed. Its prevalence is also increasing, with an increase in 13.5% from 2005 to 2007. There were 1.6 million new cases of diabetes diagnosed in people aged 20 years and older in 2007. It is also a common cause of mortality, as it was the fifth leading cause of death in 2005, accounting for 233,619 deaths.[1]

The economic impact of diabetes in the United States is quite substantial. In 2007, the total annual economic cost of diabetes was approximately $174 billion. Medical expenditures totaled $116 billion, which consisted of $27 billion for directly treating diabetes, $58 billion to treat chronic diabetes-related conditions, and $31 billion for excess general costs. The indirect costs have been estimated to be as high as $58 billion, and result from increased absenteeism, reduced productivity, disease-related disability, and loss of productive capacity caused by early mortality.[1]

Diabetes is a disease that affects multiple organ systems. It has been attributed to heart disease and stroke, hypertension, blindness, renal disease, neuropathy, amputations, pregnancy complications, and sexual dysfunction. A multidisciplinary team approach is essential to increase the chances of successful patient outcomes. This collaboration includes involvement of the foot and ankle surgeon, vascular surgeon, endocrinologist, infectious disease specialist, plastic surgeon, physical therapist, orthotist, and pedorthotist.

Foot complications, including infection, are the most common reason for hospital admission in patients with diabetes mellitus in the United States and are commonly encountered by the foot and ankle surgeon.[2] Infection of the diabetic foot is a common cause of lower extremity amputation. In 2004, about 71,000 nontraumatic lower-limb amputations occurred in diabetics, which is more than 60% of all nontraumatic lower limb amputations.[3] This article reviews the pathophysiology, diagnosis, and management of diabetic infections in the foot and ankle.

Orthopedic Foot and Ankle Center, 300 Polaris Parkway, Suite 2000, Westerville, OH 43082, USA
Corresponding author. c/o Emily Stansbury.
E-mail address: ofacresearch@orthofootankle.com

Foot Ankle Clin N Am 15 (2010) 465–476
doi:10.1016/j.fcl.2010.03.006
1083-7515/10/$ – see front matter © 2010 Elsevier Inc. All rights reserved.

foot.theclinics.com

PATHOPHYSIOLOGY

Neuropathy is a common comorbidity in diabetics and plays a significant role in the development of foot ulcers and infections. The pathogenesis of neuropathy is related to hyperglycemia. Hyperglycemia leads to a complex interplay of events, including ischemic nerve injury from microvascular disease and metabolic nerve injury from abnormal metabolic function, both of which contribute to the development of neuropathy.[4,5] Risk factors for development of neuropathy include increased age, poor glycemic control, and height.[4] The severity of neuropathy seems to be related to the severity and chronicity of hyperglycemia. Thus, the poorer control of glucose levels and the longer length of duration of hyperglycemia, the more severe the levels of neuropathy.[4]

Sensory neuropathy is the most common form of neuropathy encountered in diabetics, affecting approximately 75% of patients.[5,6] Symptoms typically begin in the toes and will gradually ascend proximally. Sensory loss can be caused by large or small fiber loss. Large fiber loss affects proprioception and light touch, whereas small fiber loss affects pain and temperature perception.[5,6] A mixed large and small fiber variant often occurs, with a combination of these symptoms and findings.[5]

Autonomic neuropathy occurs in 20% to 40% of diabetics and often occurs in conjunction with sensory neuropathy.[5] Autonomic neuropathy results in loss of normal control of sweat glands in the skin, causing dry and scaly skin. Abnormalities in thermoregulation of skin temperature and loss of normal hyperemic response also occur. As a result, cracks in the skin can develop easily and allow bacteria to invade and cause infection.

Motor neuropathy causes weakness of the intrinsic muscles of the foot, leading to contracture of the toes and development of claw toe deformities. This deformity causes an increase in pressure at the dorsum of the toes and at the plantar aspect of the metatarsal heads, placing the foot at an increased risk for ulceration. Patients also often have involvement of the anterior and lateral compartments of the leg, causing weak dorsiflexion and eversion of the foot. An equinus contracture results, as the posterior compartment muscles overpower the weakened anterior and lateral muscles.[4] An equinus contracture can lead to an increase in forefoot pressures and subsequently an increased risk for future ulceration.

Neuropathy is recognized as the major factor predisposing patients to skin breakdown and the development of ulcers. Although peripheral vascular disease often coexists with neuropathy, it is related more to delayed wound healing and is not the initiating event in ulceration. Multiple risk factors for the development of a new ulcer have been described and include a history of a previous ulcer, an abnormal Neuropathy Disability score, prior treatment of the foot, inability to perceive sensation from a 10-g monofilament, diminished pulses, pedal deformities, abnormal reflexes, and advanced patient age.[7] Insulin usage, foot deformity, increased body weight, decreased vascularity, and poor vision are other risk factors.[8] Finally, the triad of neuropathy, repetitive foot trauma, and foot deformity places patients at increased risk for ulcer formation.[9]

The development of diabetic foot infection typically begins with a loss of skin integrity and subsequent progression to diabetic foot ulceration, which creates a portal of entry for bacteria into the deeper tissues of the foot. The altered immune function in diabetics may decrease the body's ability to fight off the bacteria and infection ensues. Compared with the nondiabetic population, diabetics have an 80% increased risk for cellulitis, a fourfold increased risk for osteomyelitis, and a twofold increased risk of sepsis and death resulting from infection.[10]

MICROBIOLOGY

The most important characteristic of the microbiology of diabetic foot infections is that they are frequently polymicrobial. The presence of polymicrobial flora has been reported to be as high as 83% in some studies.[11] The failure to look for multiple organisms can adversely affect treatment and outcomes. The microbiological profiles of 825 subjects with infected diabetic foot ulcers were reviewed. Of the infected diabetic ulcers, 75% had multiple organisms, with an average of 2.4 organisms per wound. Gram positive aerobic bacteria were the most common (68%), with *Staphylococcus*, *Enterococcus*, and *Streptococcus* being the most frequent organisms. Gram negative aerobes were less common (24%), with *Pseudomonas aeruginosa* and *Escherichia coli* being the most frequent. Anaerobes (6%) and fungal species (3%) were the least common organisms.[12] In a more recent study identifying the common organisms present in a group of infected diabetic foot ulcer cultures, *S aureus* was the most common pathogen isolated, present in 38% of cases, whereas *P aeruginosa* and *Proteus mirabilis* were each present in nearly 18% of cases.[13]

The presence of antibiotic resistant bacteria is an emerging problem in diabetic foot infections. In a study comparing the prevalence of methicillin resistant *Staphylococcus aureus* (MRSA) in diabetic foot ulcers from 1998 to those in 2001, the incidence of MRSA was almost double the 1998 rate.[14] Risk factors associated with the development of multidrug-resistant organisms include previous hospitalization for the same wound, the presence of osteomyelitis, and proliferative retinopathy.[15,16]

Proper culture technique is important to identify all organisms causing the infection. Aerobic and anaerobic cultures should be obtained. Culture material from deep tissues under sterile conditions should be performed and is more reliable than superficial swabs of wounds or ulcers. If osteomyelitis is suspected, biopsy from bone may be required. In a study comparing percutaneous bone biopsy to superficial swab cultures of diabetic foot ulcers in 69 subjects with osteomyelitis, culture results were identical in only 12 subjects (17.4%). These results suggest that superficial swab cultures do not reliably detect bone bacteria.[17]

CLINICAL EVALUATION

The diagnosis of infection is made clinically with the aid of diagnostic studies. Prompt diagnosis is essential to ensure success with initial treatment and prevent any complications. Therefore, the Diabetic Committee of The American Orthopaedic Foot & Ankle Society (AOFAS) recommends yearly foot examinations in diabetics and more frequent examinations in patients who are high-risk.[2]

The orthopedic assessment in patients with diabetic foot disorders should include evaluation of both extremities up to the level of the knee. This evaluation will prevent the examiner from overlooking any disorder or problem on the lesser-involved extremity. Initially, the patients' gait should be assessed, noting any gait abnormalities. The patients' shoes should be inspected, noting the wear pattern and to also identify any areas of the shoe causing increased pressure on the foot, foreign objects, and the presence of blood or other drainage.

Clinical signs and symptoms of infection include erythema, edema, warmth, and pain. The presence of purulence, a crepitant sound, or foul-smelling drainage should also be assessed. Constitutional symptoms, such as fevers and chills, general malaise, loss of appetite, and nausea and vomiting, may suggest a more serious infection. As previously stated, foot infection in diabetics is often the result of a break in the skin and development of an ulcer, creating a portal of entry for bacteria.

Evaluation of the ulcer is critical, and begins with assessment of the location, size, and depth of the ulcer, and any associated drainage, odor, erythema, and edema (**Fig. 1**). The classification of ulcers was originally described by Wagner.[18] A Grade 0 ft is a foot with intact skin, but with risk factors for future ulceration. A Grade 1 ft is a superficial ulcer in the skin only. A Grade 2 ft has a deeper ulcer with full thickness extension. A Grade 3 ft has deeper extension that includes exposed bone, abscess formation, or osteomyelitis. A Grade 4 ft has a gangrenous area of some portion of the foot. Finally, a Grade 5 ft is gangrenous over the greater percentage of the foot.[18] The presence or absence of osteomyelitis is an important determination to make. The presence of exposed bone or the ability to probe to bone in a diabetic ulcer has been shown to correlate with the presence of underlying osteomyelitis.[19,20] However, a recent meta-analysis revealed that the presence of exposed bone or a positive probe-to-bone test result is only moderately predictive of osteomyelitis.[21]

Assessment for the presence of neuropathy and protective sensation should be performed. Historically, protective sensation has been described as present if patients can perceive a 5.07-g monofilament applied perpendicular to the skin.[22] More recently it was described that the inability to perceive 4.5-g monofilament sensation beneath both first metatarsal heads indicates that patients have lost protective sensation and are at an increased risk for ulceration or undetected injury.[23]

Finally, assessment of the vascular status of the foot is also important. The main goal of the vascular examination is to determine if the ulcer or wound can heal primarily.[24] Evaluation includes palpation of the dorsalis pedis and posterior tibial pulses and capillary refill. Skin temperature is also assessed, because coolness

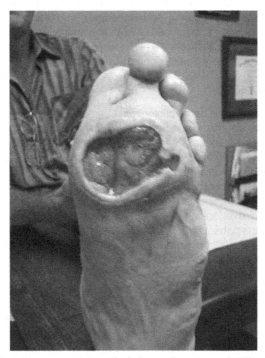

Fig. 1. Large forefoot ulcer in patient with diabetes. (*Courtesy of* William DeCarbo, D.P.M., Columbus, OH.)

may indicate decreased perfusion and warmth may indicate infection or inflammation. Thin, shiny, atrophic, and hairless skin is indicative of decreased vascularity. If any of these examination findings are abnormal, further vascular screening studies should be performed. These studies can be in the form of arterial Doppler studies, absolute toe pressures, transcutaneous oxygen measurements, or arteriography. The most common method is arterial Doppler ultrasound measurements. Wagner described that a ratio of ankle pressures to arm pressures greater than 0.45 was necessary to heal diabetic foot lesions.[18] This ratio should be used as a rough guideline, however, as calcification of the lower extremity vessels can falsely elevate the pressure readings. Examining the waveform patterns of the study can be a useful adjunct, because a monophasic waveform indicates a calcified vessel and a low potential of healing. Absolute toe pressure measurements are more reliable than ankle-brachial indices in predicting wound healing.[25] In a study comparing the two methods, Apelqvist and colleagues[25] found a healing rate of 85% in subjects with diabetic foot ulcers who had absolute toe pressures greater than 45 mmHg, whereas no subject healed primarily with an ankle pressure less than 40 mmHg. Transcutaneous oxygen measurements are also useful. A TcPO2 greater than 30 mmHg indicates adequate healing potential. However, edema, cellulitis, and venous outflow abnormalities can alter the TcPO2 reading.[26] In patients with significant vascular disease, arteriography and a consultation with a vascular surgeon may be required.

LABORATORY STUDIES

Laboratory testing for a suspected infection should include a complete blood count with differential, an erythrocyte sedimentation rate (ESR), and a C-reactive protein (CRP). In addition to aiding in diagnosis, an ESR and CRP can also be useful for monitoring the response to therapy. A normal white blood cell count (WBC) can often be found in acute osteomyelitis of the foot, as demonstrated by Armstrong and colleagues.[27] In their study, 54% of subjects with acute osteomyelitis of the foot secondary to neuropathic ulceration had a normal white blood cell count, whereas the ESR was elevated in 96% of subjects.

IMAGING STUDIES

Standard three-view, weight-bearing radiographs of the foot are important in the initial evaluation. Radiographs should be examined for the presence of periosteal reaction, boney erosions, or the presence of gas in the soft tissues. Plain radiographic changes often lag behind the onset of boney involvement by 10 to 14 days.[28,29] However, these initial radiographs can also act as a baseline for comparison with future radiographs.

The presence of hypertrophic new bone formation and fragmentation can often be seen in osteomyelitis and Charcot arthropathy,[30] which can present as a diagnostic challenge to the clinician. Elevating the foot for 5 to 10 minutes above the level of the heart can help distinguish between the two processes (**Fig. 2**). If an underlying infection is present, the erythema will not recede, whereas in a Charcot joint the underlying rubor will recede.[30] Labeled WBC scans can also be useful in this situation. Multiple studies have shown that labeled WBC scans are highly specific for deep infection and osteomyelitis.[31–33] Although very effective, disadvantages of labeled WBC include long preparation time, low count rates resulting in poor spatial resolution, the absence of boney landmarks, and their high cost.[32]

Lastly, MRI is very helpful in diagnosing diabetic infections, abscesses, and osteomyelitis. Advantages are that it provides superior anatomic detail and allows for the ability to identify any areas of soft tissue inflammation, abscess formation, sinus tracts,

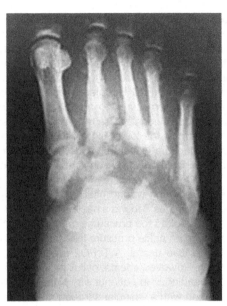

Fig. 2. Radiograph demonstrating erosive changes in the midfoot. Elevating the foot for 5 to 10 minutes above the level of the heart can help distinguish between Charcot arthropathy and osteomyelitis. (*Courtesy of* William DeCarbo, D.P.M., Columbus, OH.)

and early marrow edema in bone that is seen in osteomyelitis.[34] A recent meta-analysis assessing various imaging tests for diagnosing osteomyelitis of the foot in diabetics revealed MRI to be the most accurate test.[21]

Currently there is no imaging study that is 100% effective and occasionally a bone biopsy is necessary to make a diagnosis of osteomyelitis.

TREATMENT

The treatment of diabetic foot infections requires a multidisciplinary team approach consisting of surgeons, infectious disease specialists, endocrinologists, and the foot and ankle specialist. This type of team approach improves outcomes in the treatment of such foot and ankle infections.[35–37]

Antibiotic therapy is essential in the management of diabetic foot infections. Initial antibiotic selection should be empiric. This selection can range from coverage for Staphylococcus or Streptococcus in the treatment of simple cellulitis to more broad-spectrum antibiotic coverage for more severe infections. As previously discussed, diabetic foot infections are frequently polymicrobial. Therefore, broad-spectrum coverage should target Gram positive and Gram negative organisms, and aerobes and anaerobes. Numerous antibiotic agents and combinations are available for empiric therapy. These can include penicillin/beta-lactam inhibitors, cephalosporins, clindamycin, fluoroquinolones, imipenem, and linezolid. Diamantopoulos and colleagues[11] used initial empiric antibiotic therapy with ciprofloxacin and clindamycin in 84 subjects with severe diabetic foot infections and found that this combination was effective against 94% of the in vitro isolated organisms. In their study, Abdulrazak and colleagues[13] showed that imipenem, meropenem, and cefepime were the most effective agents against gram-negative organism, whereas vancomycin was the most effective agent for gram-positive organisms. No single agent or combination, however, has been proven to be 100% effective.[38] Once final cultures and sensitivities are available, they can be used to guide definitive therapy.

Duration of antimicrobial therapy can vary. For deep infections that do not involve bone, a 14-day course of antibiotic therapy is often adequate. However, in deep infections that involve bone or if the infected tissue has not been removed surgically, 6 to 12 weeks of antibiotic therapy is necessary.[39]

Although antibiotic therapy can result in remission of deep infections, surgical debridement is often necessary to fully eradicate deep infection and osteomyelitis (**Fig. 3**). Foot salvage should be the primary goal.[40] Indications for surgical treatment of diabetic foot infections include a draining sinus, an infected non-granulating ulcer, abscess formation, osteomyelitis, exposed nonviable tissue, and exposed cartilage or boney surface.[30] Early surgical intervention with antibiotic therapy significantly improves patient outcomes. A retrospective study of 112 subjects compared subjects with diabetes with deep foot infections treated by intravenous antibiotics with no surgical debridement during the first 3 days of hospitalization to a group who received intravenous antibiotics and surgical debridement within the first 3 days of hospitalization. The authors found a significantly higher incidence of above ankle amputation in the group treated without early surgical intervention – a 92% compared with a 2% rate of amputation.[41] Faglia and colleagues[42] also showed a higher amputation rate in subjects with deep-space foot infections who were treated with a delay in surgical debridement compared with a group treated with early surgical debridement.

Patients displaying systemic signs and symptoms of infection (fevers, chills, tachycardia, hypotension) should be treated with urgent surgical debridement. Necrotizing fasciitis is a rapidly spreading soft-tissue infection of the superficial and deep fascia that has been associated with diabetes mellitus. Patients present with severe pain, signs of systemic toxicity, and multiorgan failure. It should be treated as a surgical emergency, with prompt recognition and radical debridement of devitalized tissue to save the limbs and lives of patients, because mortality can be high with this disease.[43]

Mild infections generally involve superficial ulcerations with associated cellulitis. There are no signs or symptoms of systemic toxicity, and no boney or joint

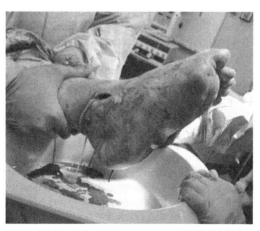

Fig. 3. Diabetic foot with abscess undergoing surgical irrigation and debridement. (*Courtesy of* William DeCarbo, D.P.M., Columbus, OH.)

involvement. These can usually be treated in the outpatient setting. Treatment requires serial debridement of the ulcer, removing all necrotic tissue and callus formation and local wound care. Appropriate antibiotic coverage is frequently used as initial therapy. After initial debridement, the patients are followed weekly or biweekly for repeat debridement until complete healing occurs.

Moderate to severe infections typically involve the deeper tissues and generally require hospitalization and surgical debridement. If an abscess is suspected, MRI is useful to localize and determine its extent and to aid in preoperative planning. Abscesses of the foot must be drained. Longitudinal incisions allow for easier extension of incisions and plantar incisions should be avoided if possible.[44]

In cases of established osteomyelitis, intravenous antibiotics rarely eradicate the infection and surgical debridement is often required. The surgical debridement of osteomyelitis involves resecting the infected bone and debridement of all surrounding necrotic and infected tissue. Wide excision of necrotic and infected bone with 5 mm or greater clearance reduces the risk for recurrent infection compared with groups in which marginal resection (<5 mm of clearance) was obtained.[45] However, it is important to try to preserve as much bone as possible to maintain stability and function of the foot.

Most cases of osteomyelitis of the foot occur in the forefoot because this is the most common site of ulceration. Debridement is typically performed through an incision away from the ulcer or draining wound, and not through the infected wound itself, which allows for avoidance of plantar incisions. The second wound can be closed loosely to allow drainage, provided the ulcer is also debrided.[40]

Osteomyelitis of the digits is treated with amputation of the affected toe. It is not always necessary to amputate toes at the level of the metatarsophalangeal joints because this can cause varus or valgus drifting of adjacent toes. If the extent of osteomyelitis allows, partial amputation of the toe should be performed so that the stump can serve as a spacer between the toes and prevent any drift of the adjacent toes.[26]

The metatarsal heads are a very common site of osteomyelitis because they are the site of frequent ulcerations of the foot. Metatarsal head resection in this instance is the treatment of choice. If more than one metatarsal head is affected and transfer lesions develop, resection of all lesser metatarsal heads or a transmetatarsal amputation should be considered if conservative treatment fails.[40] If the osteomyelitis extends more proximal in the metatarsal, ray amputation or transmetatarsal amputation is required. After appropriate surgical treatment, appropriate footwear and inserts should be worn to prevent the risk for recurrent ulceration and infection.

Osteomyelitis of the midfoot typically occurs in patients with Charcot arthropathy with midfoot deformity. The prominent boney structures cause increased pressure on the skin and subsequent ulceration, which can lead to deep infection. Exostectomy of the boney prominence through a separate incision with debridement of the ulcer is recommended.[46] It is important to balance removing enough bone to decrease the pressure on the soft tissues while preserving enough bone to maintain stability and function. The presence of osteomyelitis at the base of the fifth metatarsal should alert the foot and ankle surgeon of a possible hindfoot varus deformity, which should be addressed at the time of debridement to prevent ulcer recurrence.

In the hindfoot, osteomyelitis is difficult to manage because of its thin and immobile skin with little soft tissue available for coverage. Amputation was a common treatment as a result. More recently, partial or total calcanectomy has been described as a treatment method for osteomyelitis of the posterior portion of the calcaneus.[47–49] The procedure allows for eradication of infection, soft-tissue relaxation from the boney resection to allow for a tension-free closure, preservation of the limb, and functional ambulation. A longitudinal posterior incision is made with an elliptical excision of the ulcer. The Achilles is split longitudinally for exposure while preserving its attachments with the distal plantar tissues. All infected bone and nonviable tissue is resected and the wound can be closed primarily.[47–49] Failure of partial or total calcanectomy usually leads to a below-the-knee amputation.

After thorough debridement, if there is adequate soft-tissue coverage and the wound is clean, primary wound closure can be performed. If, however, there is any question that soft-tissue infection remains, multiple debridements may be required. Vacuum-assisted closure can be used in this situation and can be a useful adjunct in treatment. It expedites healing of these wounds and may even decrease the need for repeat debridements.[50,51]

Despite attempts at limb salvage, amputations are common in diabetics. The rate of amputation is 10 times more common in diabetics than in the nondiabetic population, with more than 60% of all nontraumatic lower-extremity amputations performed in diabetics.[1] Also, following an amputation, 30% of amputees will undergo an amputation of their contralateral limb within 3 years and two thirds will die within 5 years.[52] The different levels of amputation include partial-digital, digital, ray resection, transmetatarsal, Chopart, Symes, below-the-knee, and above-the-knee. Preoperatively, it is important to assess the quality of tissue, extent of infection, and the vascular status and wound-healing potential of the limb. Such factors will aid the surgeon in determining the level of amputation. A serum albumin level of 3.0 g/dL and a total lymphocyte count of greater than 1500 correlate with good wound-healing potential.[26] An important aspect to consider in determining level of amputation is that energy consumption following an amputation is inversely proportional to the length of the residual limb.[53] Thus, the more proximal the amputation level the greater the amount of energy required during activity. Therefore, more distal limb conserving amputations are preferred when possible. Finally, patients should be reminded that because of advances in orthotics, prosthetics, and rehabilitation, positive outcomes following amputation can be achieved.

SUMMARY

Thus, diabetes mellitus is a common and increasing medical problem in the world today, with foot and ankle infections continuing to be a common complication of the disease. Thorough clinical examination with appropriate use of adjunctive laboratory and imaging studies can allow for early diagnosis and treatment, which can improve patient outcomes. Most mild infections can be treated on an outpatient basis with oral antibiotics and local debridement, whereas more severe infections require hospitalization, intravenous antibiotics, and surgical debridement to fully eradicate the infection. Despite proper treatment, amputation is still common in diabetics.

REFERENCES

1. American Diabetes Association. Diabetes statistics. Available at: http://www.diabetes.org/diabetes-statistics.jsp. Accessed October 22, 2009.
2. Pinzur MS, Slovenaki MP, Trepman E, et al. Diabetes Committee of American Orthopaedic Foot and Ankle Society. Guidelines for diabetic foot care: recommendations endorsed by the Diabetes Committee of the American Orthopaedic Foot and Ankle Society. Foot Ankle Int 2005;26:113–9.
3. Centers for disease control. Available at: http://www.cdc.gov/diabetes/pubs/pdf/ndfs_2007.pdf. Accessed October 22, 2009.
4. Bibbo C, Patel DV. Diabetic neuropathy. Foot Ankle Clin 2006;11:753–74.

5. Ross MA. Neuropathies associated with diabetes. Med Clin North Am 1993;77: 111–24.
6. Cameron NE, Eaton SE, Cotter MA, et al. Vascular factors and metabolic interactions in the pathogenesis of diabetic neuropathy. Diabetologia 2001;44:1973–88.
7. Abbott CA, Carrington AL, Ashe H, et al. The northwest diabetes foot care study: incidence of and risk factors for new diabetic foot ulceration in a community patient cohort. Diabet Med 2002;19:377–84.
8. Singh N, Armstrong DG, Lipsky BA. Preventing foot ulcers in patients with diabetes. JAMA 2005;293:217–28.
9. Reiber GE, Smith DG, Wallace C, et al. Effect of therapeutic footwear on foot reulceration in patients with diabetes: a randomized control trial. JAMA 2002;287: 2552–8.
10. Shah BR, Hux JE. Quantifying the risk of infectious diseases for people with diabetes. Diabetes Care 2003;26:510–3.
11. Diamantopoulos EJ, Haritos D, Yfandi G, et al. Management and outcome of severe diabetic foot infections. Exp Clin Endocrinol Diabetes 1998;106:346–52.
12. Ge Y, MacDonald H, Lipsky B, et al. Microbiological profile of infected diabetic foot ulcers. Diabet Med 2002;19:1032–4.
13. Abdulrazak A, Bitar ZI, Al-Shamali AA, et al. Bacteriological study of diabetic foot infections. J Diabetes Complications 2005;19:138–41.
14. Dang CN, Prasad YD, Boulton AJ, et al. Methicillin-resistant *Staphylococcus aureus* in the diabetic foot clinic: a worsening problem. Diabet Med 2003;20: 159–61.
15. Harteman-Heurtier A, Robert J, Jacqueminet S, et al. Diabetic foot ulcer and multidrug resistant organisms: risk factors and impact. Diabet Med 2004;21:710–5.
16. Richard JL, Sotto A, Jourdan N, et al. Risk factors and healing impact of multidrug-resistant bacteria in diabetic foot ulcers. Diabetes Metab 2008;34:363–9.
17. Senneville E, Melliez H, Beltrand E, et al. Culture of percutaneous bone biopsy specimens for diagnosis of diabetic ulcer osteomyelitis: concordance with ulcer swab cultures. Clin Infect Dis 2006;42:57–62.
18. Wagner F. A classification and treatment program for diabetic, neuropathic and dysvascular foot problems. Instr Course Lect 1979;28:143–65.
19. Grayson ML, Gibbons GW, Balogh K, et al. Probing to bone in infected pedal ulcers. A clinical sign of underlying osteomyelitis in diabetic patients. JAMA 1995;273:721–3.
20. Newman LG, Waller J, Paletro CJ, et al. Unsuspected osteomyelitis in diabetic foot ulcers: diagnosis and monitoring by leukocyte scanning with indium in 111 oxyquinoline. JAMA 1991;266:1246–51.
21. Dinh MT, Abad CL, Safdar N. Diagnostic accuracy of the physical examination and imaging tests for osteomyelitis underlying diabetic foot ulcers: meta-analysis. Clin Infect Dis 2008;47:519–27.
22. Birk JA, Sims DS. Plantar sensory threshold in the ulcerative foot. Lepr Rev 1986; 57:261–7.
23. Saltzman CL, Rashid R, Hayes A, et al. 4.5 gram monofilament sensation beneath both first metatarsal heads indicates protective foot sensation in diabetic patients. J Bone Joint Surg Am 2004;86-A:717–23.
24. Shapiro SA, Stansberry KB, Hill MA, et al. Normal blood flow response and vasomotion in the diabetic Charcot foot. J Diabetes Complications 1998;12:147–53.
25. Apelqvist J, Castenfors J, Larson J, et al. Prognostic value of systolic ankle and toe blood pressure levels in outcome of diabetic foot ulcer. Diabetes Care 1989; 12:373–8.

26. Philbin TM, Berlet GC, Lee TH. Lower-extremity amputations in association with diabetes mellitus. Foot Ankle Clin 2006;11:791–804.
27. Armstrong DG, Lavery LA, Sariaya M, et al. Leukocytosis is a poor indicator of osteomyelitis of the foot in diabetes mellitus. J Foot Ankle Surg 1996;35:280–3.
28. Lipsky BA. Osteomyelitis of the foot in diabetic patients. Clin Infect Dis 1997;25: 1318–26.
29. Longmaid HE, Kruskal JB. Imaging infections in diabetic patients. Infect Dis Clin North Am 1995;9:163–82.
30. Brodsky JW, Schneidler C. Diabetic foot infections. Orthop Clin North Am 1991; 22:473–89.
31. Johnson JE, Kennedy EJ, Shereff MJ, et al. Prospective study of bone, indium 111-labeled white blood cell, and gallium-67 scanning for the evaluation of osteomyelitis in the diabetic foot. Foot Ankle Int 1996;17:10–6.
32. Maurer AH, Millmond SH, Knight LC, et al. Infection in diabetic osteoarthropathy: use of indium-labeled leukocytes for diagnosis. Radiology 1986;161:221–5.
33. Splittgerber GF, Spiegelhoff DR, Buggy BP. Combined leukocyte and bone imaging used to evaluate diabetic osteoarthropathy and osteomyelitis. Clin Nucl Med 1989;14:156–60.
34. Stapp MD, Hodos MJ, Austin JH Jr. Current trends in the management of foot and ankle infections. J Foot Ankle Surg 2004;43(Suppl):1–23.
35. Holstein PE, Sorenson S. Limb salvage experience in a multidisciplinary diabetic foot unit. Diabetes care 1999;22(Suppl 2):B97–103.
36. Dargis V, Pantelejava O, Jonushaite A, et al. Benefits of a multidisciplinary approach in the management of recurrent diabetic foot ulceration in Lithuania. Diabetes Care 1999;22:1428–31.
37. Frykberg RG. Team approach toward lower extremity amputation in diabetes. J Am Podiatr Med Assoc 1997;87:305–12.
38. Lipsky BA. Medical treatment of diabetic foot infections. Clin Infect Dis 2004;39: S101–114.
39. Tan JS, File TM Jr. Diagnosis and treatment of diabetic foot infections. Baillieres Best Pract Res Clin Rheumatol 1999;13:149–61.
40. Brodsky JW. The diabetic foot. In: Coughlin MJ, Mann RA, Saltzman CL, editors. Surgery of the foot and ankle. 8th edition. Philadelphia: Mosby; 2007. p. 1281–369.
41. Tan JS, Friedman NM, Hazelton-Miller C, et al. Can aggressive treatment of diabetic foot infections reduce the need for above-ankle amputation? Clin Infect Dis 1996;23:286–91.
42. Faglia E, Clerici G, Caminiti M, et al. The role of early surgical debridement and revascularization in patients with diabetes and deep foot space abscess: retrospective review of 106 patients with diabetes. J Foot Ankle Surg 2006;45: 220–6.
43. Childers BJ, Potyonay LD, Nachreiner R, et al. Necrotizing fasciitis: a 14 year retrospective study of 163 consecutive patients. Am Surg 2002;68:109–16.
44. Shank CF, Feibel JB. Osteomyelitis in the diabetic foot: diagnosis and management. Foot Ankle Clin 2006;11:775–89.
45. Simpson AH, Deakin M, Latham JM. Chronic osteomyelitis: the effect of the extent of surgical resection on infection-free survival. J Bone Joint Surg Br 2001;83: 403–7.
46. van der Ven A, Chapman CB, Bowker JH. Charcot neuroarthropathy of the foot and ankle. J Am Acad Orthop Surg 2009;17:562–71.
47. Bollinger M, Thordarson DB. Partial calcanectomy: an alternative to below knee amputation. Foot Ankle Int 2002;23:927–32.

48. Baumhauer JF, Fraga CJ, Gould JS, et al. Total calcanectomy for the treatment of chronic calcaneal osteomyelitis. Foot Ankle Int 1998;19:849–55.

49. Crandall RC, Wagner FW Jr. Partial and total calcanectomy: a review of thirty-one consecutive cases over a ten-year period. J Bone Joint Surg Am 1981;63:152–5.

50. Armstrong DG, Lavery LA. Negative pressure therapy after partial diabetic foot amputation: a multicenter, randomized controlled trial. Lancet 2006;366:1704–10.

51. Mendonca DA, Cosker T, Makwana NK. Vacuum-assisted closure to aid wound healing in foot and ankle surgery. Foot Ankle Int 2005;26:761–6.

52. Philbin TM, Leyes M, Sferra JJ, et al. Orthotic and prosthetic devices in partial foot amputation. Foot Ankle Clin 2001;6:215–28.

53. Smith DG, Ehde DM, Legro MW, et al. Phantom limb, residual limb, and back pain after lower extremity amputations. Clin Orthop Relat Res 1999;361:29–38.

The Infected Calcaneus

Tomiko Fukuda, MD[a], Verrabdhadra Reddy, MD[b],
Amy Jo Ptaszek, MD[c,d],*

KEYWORDS

• Infection • Calcaneus • Angiosomes

Infections in and around the calcaneus can be quite challenging for the patients and physicians involved. These infections arise because of multiple potential etiologies, including chronic pressure, trauma, and postsurgical wound-healing complications. The impediments to healing can be equally as diverse depending on the patients' comorbidities, such as smoking, diabetes, and open injury.[1] In this article the authors review the anatomy of the calcaneus and surrounding soft tissue, patient risk factors, and various treatment options that can be used through a multidisciplinary approach. The common limiting factor for most of these patients is the delicate soft-tissue envelope, and occasionally, the lack thereof. The ultimate goal is an infection-free limb with durable soft-tissue coverage and maximal maintenance of function.[2]

ANATOMY
Bone

As the strongest bone in the foot, the calcaneus has a unique role in gait because it accepts axial load during heel strike then later transmits forces to the forefoot during push off.[3] The calcaneus has four articular surfaces. The anterior, middle, and posterior facets that articulate with the talus allow heal inversion and eversion, which thereby enable accommodation of uneven surfaces. The calcaneal cuboid articulation plays an important role anteriorly in supporting the lateral column.[4] The sustentaculum tali, which projects anteromedially from the sulcus calcanei, supports the talar neck above via the anterior and middle facets; it also allows passage of the flexor hallucis longus below and is stabilized medially by the talocalcaneal ligaments.[4] The sulcus calcanei forms the inferior border of the medial tarsal canal and the lateral sinus tarsi, which contains the interosseus ligament connecting the talus and calcaneus. The Achilles tendon inserts on the posterior tubercle, whereas the medial and lateral processes provide origins for the abductor hallucis and abductor digiti quinti muscles, respectively.[5] The lateral surface also has grooves for the traversal of the peroneal

[a] Fondren Orthopaedic Group LLC, 10223 Broadway Street, Suite A, Pearland, TX 77584, USA
[b] Austin Orthopaedics, 4316 James Casey Street, Austin, Texas 78745, USA
[c] Department of Orthopaedic Surgery, The University of Chicago, Chicago, IL, USA
[d] Illinois Bone and Joint Institute, LTD, 2401 Ravine Way, Glenview, IL 60025, USA
* Corresponding author. Illinois Bone and Joint, 2401 Ravine Way, Glenview, IL 60025.
E-mail address: amytoe@hotmail.com

Foot Ankle Clin N Am 15 (2010) 477–486
doi:10.1016/j.fcl.2010.04.002
1083-7515/10/$ – see front matter © 2010 Elsevier Inc. All rights reserved.

foot.theclinics.com

tendons with the peroneal tubercle separating the peroneus brevis above from the peroneus longus below at this level. The thickest cortex can be seen along the superior neck on a lateral radiograph and marks the crucial angle of Gissane,[6] which normally ranges from 120° to 145°. The relation of the top of posterior facet to the superior aspect of the posterior tuberosity and top of the anterior process of the calcaneus can also be evaluated on a lateral radiograph and delineates Bohler's angle, which is normally 25° to 40°.[7]

Vascular

The concept of angiosomes was popularized by Taylor and Palmer in 1987 after serial cadaveric arterial injections to determine regions of direct perfusion and anastomoses between such territories.[8,9] An angiosome is a region of tissue supplied by a named artery. They define the anastomoses between these angiosomes as choke vessels, which are more commonly known as watershead areas.[10] In 1997, Taylor and colleagues further examined the angiosomes within the leg, which enhanced our insight into potential flap options and strategies for surgical incisions.[8]

The peroneal artery plays a prominent role in calcaneal wound healing as it supplies the lateral aspect of the ankle and hindfoot via the calcaneal and anterior perforating branches. When evaluating the ankle and foot, there are predictable interconnections between the three main arteries: the posterior tibial (PT); anterior tibial (AT); and peroneal (P), which can provide back-up flow should any major vessel be disrupted. At the Lisfranc joint, the PT and AT connect via the lateral plantar (PT) and dorsalis pedis (DP) (AT). There are potentially three communicating branches between the posterior tibial and peroneal arteries: 5 to 7 cm above the ankle, near the ankle, and the Achilles insertion. The lateral malleolar branch off the tibialis anterior artery also connects with the perforating anterior branch off the peroneal artery. The venous drainage is via the lesser saphenous vein, which accompanies the calcaneal artery. The glabrous junction marks the transition between the lateral calcaneal artery (P) and medial calcaneal artery (PT) angiosomes. By making the incision at the junction of these angiosomes, blood flow is maximized to the healing surgical wound.[10] Before considering any flap coverage in these patients, it is important to be cognizant of the vascular status of the limb.

RISKS FOR WOUND HEALING
Operatively Treated Calcaneal Fractures

Folk and colleagues[1] looked at early wound complications in 190 operatively treated calcaneal fractures and found a 25% wound-complication rate with 21% requiring surgical treatment. They found the predictive variables in their study were smoking (37 out of 118 patients; $P = .03$; relative risk [RR] = 1.2); diabetes (7 out of 9; $P = .02$; RR = 3.4); and open injuries (13 out of 18 fractures; $P<.0001$; RR = 2.8).

Abidi and colleagues[11] also looked at wound healing risk factors in 63 subjects with 64 calcaneus fractures that underwent open reduction and internal fixation. They found a higher incidence of wound complications in those closed via a single-layer technique as opposed to the double-layer technique used in subjects later in their series (58% vs 28%; $P<.04$). The single-layer technique consisted of alternating horizontal and vertical mattress sutures. The double-layer technique added a deep layer consisting of interrupted 2–0 PDS or 0 Dexon sutures that were each tagged and tied after all were placed. They also found that smoking ($P<.05$) and body mass index ($P<.01$) positively correlated with delayed wound healing. Use of a drain did not significantly correlate with a decrease in wound complications, but 89% of their wounds were drained; therefore, this may have been secondary to sample size.[11] Looking at this same subject population, Shuler and colleagues[12] reviewed the pre- and postoperative radiographs and found that all were anatomically reduced, but they found a trend toward increased wound complications in subjects who required a greater correction in Bohler's angle.

Open Calcaneal Fractures

Though much less common, open calcaneus fractures are known to carry a higher risk for infection. Heier and colleagues[13] reported a 37% infection rate in 43 open calcaneal fractures treated, with 19% developing osteomyelitis. They experienced an increasing risk for infection with an escalating Gustillo-Anderson grade of injury with a 50% (13 out of 26) infection rate in grade III open calcaneal fractures, which corresponded with 27% osteo (7 out of 26). In the grade IIIB open fractures, 10 out of 13 became infected and 6 out of 13 developed osteomyelitis, which led to 3 out of 13 proceeding to amputation. They supported open reduction and internal fixation of grade I and II injuries with medial wounds. They also recommended that, after aggressive debridement, internal fixation of non-medial grade II and III injuries should be minimized, delayed, or avoided and early coverage should be obtained for type IIIB wounds.[13]

Benirschke and Kramer[14,15] reported a 7.7% serious infection rate in their series of 39 open calcaneus fractures as compared with 1.8% in their series of 341 closed fractures. In their subject population, the largest determinant of wound infection was subject noncompliance, which was seen in one 1 of 3 of their infected cases. They did not see an increase in infection in their subjects with diabetes.

Aldridge and colleagues[16] reviewed 19 subjects treated for open calcaneal fractures. Their average number of procedures per open fractured calcaneus was 2.3 (range 1–5). They found that 5 of 19 required soft-tissue coverage. All Gustillo-Anderson grade I wounds healed without incident (5 out of 5). Of the grade II fractures, 13% (1 out of 8) developed a superficial infection that required irrigation and debridement along with intravenous antibiotics. Of the grade III fractures, 5 out of 6 required flap coverage and 17% (1 out of 6) went on to below knee amputation after developing a chronic draining osteomyelitis that was not responsive to debridement.[16]

Thornton and colleagues[17] presented a treatment protocol based on wound location and size. Using this protocol in 31 open calcaneal fractures, they experienced a 29% wound complication rate. Initial wound size greater than 4 cm correlated with an increased complication rate. In their series, 50% (2 out of 4) of the lateral traumatic wounds developed complications. According to their protocol, each subject received appropriate antibiotics and operative debridement at presentation and then every 24 to 48 hours until clean. With each debridement, they attempted to close the wound. If unable to approximate the skin, they performed an open reduction through the traumatic wound to restore the hindfoot alignment and Bohler's angle while reducing the posterior facet. They held their reductions with 2.0 mm smooth Steinmann pins. If necessary, these pins gained purchase into the talar body through the posterior facet. These pins were left in place for 6 weeks. If the wound was closable and stable, then an open reduction with internal fixation was performed through an extended lateral approach, using the no-touch technique for retraction of their full-thickness flaps. Of the stable wounds that were treated with open reduction and internal fixation, 27% (5 out of 18) developed wound complications.[17]

Chronic Pressure-Related Calcaneal Wounds

Heel wounds are most commonly associated with diabetic peripheral neuropathy, but can also be associated with any other condition that prevents patients from either feeling or controlling the pressure to their heels. These less common etiologies include patients with a history of stroke, traumatic brain injury, or spinal cord injury, to name a few. According to the American Diabetes Associate, there are approximately 20.8 million diabetics in the United States, which is 7% of the population. They estimate that one-third of these people are currently undiagnosed. When a diabetic foot wound probes to the bone, it correlates with osteomyelitis approximately 85% of the time (**Fig. 1**).[2] In these patients, education and extensive clinical support are important to prevent any worsening or recurrence of these wounds. Without eliminating the excessive pressure, most treatments will predictably fail.[2]

CLINICAL EVALUATION

There are essentially two main etiologies for calcaneal osteomyelitis or surrounding wound infection: posttraumatic versus those related to chronic pressure. The posttraumatic can be divided into postsurgical, which includes wound dehiscence, acute infection, chronic infection, and open wounds acquired at time of injury. The chronic pressure wounds are usually neuropathic in etiology and are often associated with diabetes and polymicrobial infection. All patients should undergo a comprehensive clinical evaluation in addition to a review of their medical history. The sensory examination should include a 5.07 Semmes-Weinstein filament, which corresponds to 10 g of pressure. If unable to feel this filament, patients lack sufficient protective sensation.[2]

The degree of edema, erythema, and dimensions of any wounds should be assessed and documented. Erythema can be distinguished from dependant rubor by elevation of the leg. The DP and posterior tibial pulses should be checked with a Doppler if non-palpable. Ankle to brachial indexes (ABI) for the DP and PT should be accessed. ABI greater than 0.45 is necessary for predictable wound healing. In patients with severe arterial calcification, the arteries may be non-compressible, which makes ABIs unreliable. If vascular status is at all in question, arterial blood flow studies with toe pressures should be ordered and a vascular evaluation obtained. Toe pressure less than 30 mmHg indicates distal ischemia. Triphasic or biphasic arterial waveforms have better healing potential than monophasic patterns. If revascularization is necessary, patients must also be medically optimized. If severe medical comorbidities preclude revascularization, patients would not be a candidate for flap coverage.[2]

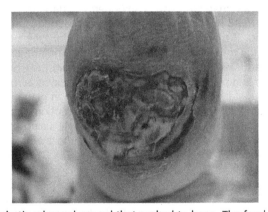

Fig. 1. Chronic diabetic calcaneal wound that probed to bone. The focal osteomyelitis was successfully treated with partial calcanectomy.

LABORATORY STUDIES

As a baseline in the workup of possible osteomyelitis, a complete blood count with differential, erythrocyte sedimentation rate (ESR), and C-reactive protein (CRP) should be checked. CRP is the most accurate indicator of osteomyelitis. It starts to elevate at 6 hours, peaks at 2 days, and normalizes in approximately 1 week after appropriate treatment is initiated. ESR can be sensitive, but lacks specificity as it becomes elevated in the presence of fracture and other inflammatory states. ESR peaks in 3 to 5 days after the start of an infectious process, and it takes approximately 3 weeks to normalize after appropriate treatment. Leukocytosis and elevated neutrophil count are suggestive of infection, but nonspecific for osteomyelitis.[18]

In addition to markers of inflammation, it is important to assess the nutritional status and glucose control if patients are diabetic. Total lymphocyte count greater than 1500 is important for wound healing potential as is an albumin greater than 3.0 g per deciliter. Hemoglobin A1C is also a helpful indicator of baseline glycemic control.[2] If patients require hospitalization, blood culture, and if necessary, bone cultures should be obtained prior to the administration of antibiotics.

IMAGING STUDIES

Radiographs should be obtained for all patients to assess radiographic evidence of osteomyelitis in addition to evaluating reduction/fixation and degree of fracture healing. It takes approximately 3 weeks for osteomyelitis to become present on plain radiographs.[2] MRI can provide earlier detection of osteomyelitis, though it is of limited utility in an instrumented calcaneus because of artifact.

Nuclear medicine imaging uses radionucleotides to better understand active physiologic changes involving inflammation and bone turnover. In the presence of osteomyelitis, a [99m]Technetium phosphonate 3- phase bone scan will demonstrate increase uptake in the initial blood flow and blood pool phases, but more importantly, it will maintain the uptake in images 2 to 4 hours post-injection. In contrast, soft-tissue infection should only demonstrate increased uptake in the initial two images. A second delayed static image can be obtained 24 hours post-injection for additional contrast of the bone uptake to the background.[19] Tagged Leukocyte scanning with indium 111 or ^{99m}Tc hexamethyl propylene amine oxine can be added to the bone scan to enhance the specificity; with images obtained 24 hours and 3 to 4 hours post-injection, respectively.

Palestro and colleagues[20] looked at the use of ^{99m}Tc labeled monoclonal anti-granulocyte antibody, Indium 111,and ^{99m}Tc three-phase bone scans in the evaluation of 25 diabetic foot wounds. They found osteomyelitis in 10 of 25 subjects. They did not find statistically significant difference results between the ^{99m}Tc labeled antibodies and the Indium 111 scans, but both were more specific and accurate than the three-phase bone scan.[20]

WOUND ISSUES AND TREATMENT OPTIONS
Inability to Achieve Primary Wound Closure

A tension-free primary closure may be difficult or impossible to obtain in patients with severe shortening or delay exceeding 2 weeks because of soft-tissue contracture. Rather than risking likely dehiscence by over tightening the deep sutures, a plastic surgeon should be made available to assist with closure.[10] Alternatively, a vacuum assisted closure (V.A.C.) (KCI, San Antonia, TX, USA) dressing can be placed and delay primary closure versus a split thickness skin graft (STSG) on a later date. If viable, the abductor digiti minimi and abductor hallucis flaps may be used for lateral or medial wounds respectively, if the wound gap is less than 1cm in width; both would be augmented with STSG.[10] For defects between 1 and 2 cm, patients may benefit from a V.A.C. dressing to shrink the wound versus a fasciocutaneous or muscular flap. Any large gap with exposed hardware will require muscle coverage, either rotational or free augmented by STSG.[10]

Acute Partial Wound Dehiscence

With the L-shaped lateral approach, partial thickness wound dehiscence or edge necrosis can appear predictably at the wound apex. This dehiscence may occur as late as 4 weeks postoperatively depending on patient compliance and their other medical comorbidities.[21] At the first sign of wound dehiscence, subtalar motion exercises should be halted to prevent further wound progression.[22] In the absence of any fluctuant drainage or exposed hardware, these wounds can be treated with oral antibiotics and local wound care, which may include whirlpool, wet to dry dressing changes, and continued elevation.[3] Though the clear mechanism of action is still unclear, the wound V.A.C. can also be used to enhance the development of granulation tissue, theoretically, by creating a hypobaric environment for the wound, which decreases edema, removes inhibitory factors, and enhances angiogenesis.[23,24]

Acute Full Thickness Wound Dehiscence

Wounds that continue to drain serous fluid and appear erythematous, despite oral antibiotics and wound care, must be surgically explored and debrided. If at any point a wound appears fluctuant or shows any purulent drainage, then urgent surgical debridement is required. If the area of infection seems contained and superficial, the hardware can be retained after thorough debridement and patients should receive a 6-week course of intravenous antibiotics (**Fig. 2**).[22] If there is any evidence of diffuse osteomyelitis, the hardware and affected bone should be removed.[22] The wound V.A.C. can also be used in these wounds to shrink the remaining wound and enhance the healing environment.[25] The use of a wound V.A.C. has the potential to decrease the degree of coverage required by our plastic surgery colleagues.[23]

CHRONIC OSTEOMYELITIS

Once osteomyelitis is recognized, adequate debridement is the cornerstone of treatment. In the setting of diffuse osteomyelitis, any internal fixation should be removed at the time of initial debridement.[22] Depending on the extent of medullary involvement and the condition of the surrounding soft-tissue envelope, the spectrum of treatment can have significant variation in complexity. If a large cavitary lesion is left post-debridement, as is common with posttraumatic osteomyelitis, options include antibiotic-impregnated polymethyl methacrylate (PMMA) beads that can be placed and later removed, tobramycin-impregnated calcium sulfate pellets,[14,26] or filling the defect with a muscular or fascial flap to enhance perfusion.[10,27–29] These cavitary lesions invariably need flap coverage; therefore, early inclusion of the plastic surgeon in the treatment is important.[2,10,30] As with all limb salvage procedures, the vascularity of the limb must be evaluated and optimized prior to any definitive plan for the treatment.[2] Any wound that requires serial debridements can be temporarily covered with antibiotic-impregnated PMMA beads if cavitary, or a silver ion sheet if flatter. Both can help to decrease bacterial count if contained in an occlusive dressing between debridements.[2] Once the wound appears clean, a wound V.A.C. can be used while awaiting plastics coverage.[23,25]

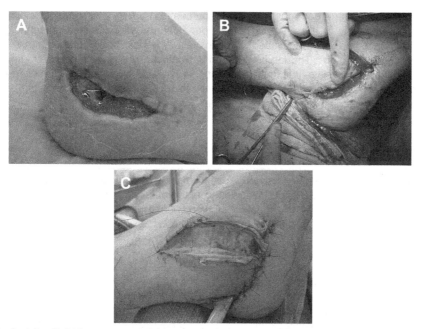

Fig. 2. (*A*) Full thickness wound dehiscence with exposed hardware. (*B*) After debridement, the hardware was retained and a local rotational flap performed. (*C*) A split-thickness skin graft was placed over the flap harvest site.

If focal osteomyelitis is identified and the surrounding soft tissue is salvageable, as is the case with many diabetic wounds first treated with total contact casting, patients could be candidates for partial calcanectomy with primary wound closure. If able to maintain their heel pad, these patients have greater preservation of their ambulatory status with the use of a heel containment orthoses.[31]

Calcanectomy

Partial or subtotal calcanectomy is a treatment option for localized infection with or without soft-tissue compromise. This situation is more commonly encountered in the neuropathic population. A combination of ischemia, ulcer, trauma, or ensuing osteomyelitis may defy local conservative measures. A partial calcanectomy in select patients yields a functional alternative to below knee amputation. Although weakness and gait dysfunction are potential complications, an ankle/foot orthosis with heel filler may compensate to afford unassisted ambulation. Sufficient perfusion is absolutely necessary for healing.[32,33]

The ulcer is excised surgically. Longitudinal extension of the incisions is made proximally along the Achilles tendon and distally onto the plantar aspect of the foot. Location of the ulcer may necessitate a more eccentric approach. Enough calcaneus is excised to obtain primary closure and the extremity is splinted in equinus to avoid tension on the suture line during healing. Reattachment of the Achilles generally is not feasible thus persistent equinus deformity is not anticipated.[32,33]

Below Knee Amputation

Amputation is the salvage procedure when patients and physicians feel they have exhausted options for limb salvage. There is tremendous variability in strategies toward limb salvage depending on the resources and beliefs of the multidisciplinary team, particularly in the diabetic population. Patients with diabetes presenting to the emergency room in the United States have a 24% risk for amputation during the same hospitalization.[2] Though amputation is significantly less common in traumatic calcaneal osteomyelitis, it is import for patients with serve injuries to appreciate the potential risks, particularly with grade III open injuries, lateral wounds, smokers, and those with significant medical comorbidities.[13,16]

SOFT-TISSUE COVERAGE OPTIONS
Skin Grafts

STSGs are used for wound coverage when there is a sufficient soft-tissue bed to accept the graft. These grafts include the epidermis and a portion of the dermis. Thinner grafts are more likely to take, but also shrink more than thicker grafts. Split-thickness skin grafts are often combined with muscular flaps to achieve adequate epidermal coverage.[2]

Local Muscle Flaps

Based on the angiosomes around the foot and ankle, there are local flaps that can be rotated for wound coverage. Unfortunately, these can be unreliable in the traumatized foot; therefore, degree of swelling and perfusion must be assessed preoperatively. The abductor digiti minimi is a useful local flap for covering small defects on the lateral aspect of the ankle and hindfoot. The lateral plantar artery provides the dominant pedicle for perfusion near the lateral calcaneal tubercle. It is distally harvested near the proximal half of the fifth metatarsal through a longitudinal incision along the glabrous junction. The abductor hallucis flap is useful for medial calcaneal wounds. The medial plantar artery provides the primary pedicel proximally near its origin on the medial calcaneal tubercle.[3,10] Distally, it can be separated from its close proximity to the flexor digitorum tendon proximal to the first metatarsal phalangeal joint. In a well-perfused foot with intact peroneal and anterior tibial artery distal anastomoses, the pedicel can be lengthened by ligating the lateral plantar artery, which lets the flap rotate from the level of the posterior tibial artery.[34]

Fasciocutaneous/Neuro-fasciocutaneous Flaps

The distally based saphenous and sural neuro-fasciocutaneous flaps can be used to cover large defects. In series of 9 performed by Yildirum and colleagues,[29] these were successful in treating chronic calcaneal osteomyelitis in 8 out of 9.[27] The flap sizes in their series ranged from 8 × 12 cm to 14 × 10 cm. These flaps depend on the retrograde perfusion that accompanies the sural and saphenous nerves; therefore, the foot must be adequately perfused distally. Chen and colleagues[27] successfully used the Sural fasciomuscular cutaneous flaps to address chronic calcaneal osteomyelitis in 11 subjects with diabetes.

Free Flaps

Free flaps are an important for patients with large soft-tissue defects with an otherwise salvageable limb. Though there are flap-harvest options all over the body, it is important to match the recipient sight size and vasculature. Before flap coverage, the wound must be clean, with viable margins and a clear recipient artery and veins. The radial forearm free flap provides good coverage and its small vessels are a reasonable match for the foot, but donor site morbidity is an issue.[3] The gracilis is a useful option-but it is limited by its short pedicle. If a longer pedicle is needed, the serratus anterior and rectus abdominis are both options; the latter is slightly preferred because it is less likely to need future debulking.[10]

SUMMARY

Infections of the calcaneus can be extremely challenging to resolve. A thorough clinical examination with close follow-up is critical for any patients at risk for developing wound complications. In the diabetic population, education and prevention are essential for minimizing the frequency and severity of calcaneal infections. Open reduction and internal fixation improves outcomes in many intraarticular calcaneal fractures, but constant cognition of the condition of the delicate soft-tissue envelope can help to minimize postoperative complications. Minimizing internal fixation in patients with large soft-tissue deficits may at times be the better part of valor. When osteomyelitis is encountered, limb perfusion must be confirmed. In conjunction with thorough debridement, early soft-tissue coverage is necessary in addition to intravenous antibiotics. If limb salvage is to be achieved for some of these more extensive infections, the multidisciplinary approach is important with the buy in and commitment of all contributors, especially patients.

REFERENCES

1. Folk JW, Starr AJ, Early JS. Early wound complications of operative treatment of calcaneus fractures: analysis of 190 fractures. J Orthop Trauma 1999;13(5): 369–72.
2. McCarthy JG, Galiano R, Boutros S. Current therapy in plastic surgery. Philadelphia (PA): Elsevier/Saunders; 2006.
3. Levin LS, Nunley JA. The management of soft-tissue problems associated with calcaneal fractures. Clin Orthop Relat Res 1993;290:151–6.
4. Moore KL. Clinically oriented anatomy. The lower limb. Philadelphia (PA): Williams & Wilkins; 1992.
5. Mann RA, Coughlin MJ. Surgery of the foot & ankle. 7th edition. Philadelphia (PA): Mosby; 1999.
6. Essex-Lopresti P. The mechanism, reduction technique, and results in fractures of the os calcis. Br J Surg 1952;39:395–419.
7. Rammelt S, Zwipp H. Calcaneus fractures: facts, controversies and recent developments. Injury 2004;35(5):443–61.
8. Taylor GI, Pan WR. Angiosomes of the leg: anatomic study and clinical implications. Plast Reconstr Surg 1998;102(3):599–616 [discussion: 617–8].
9. Thomas DB, Brooks DE, Bice TG, et al. Tobramycin-impregnated calcium sulfate prevents infection in contaminated wounds. Clin Orthop Relat Res 2005;441:366–71.
10. Attinger C, Cooper P. Soft tissue reconstruction for calcaneal fractures or osteomyelitis. Orthop Clin North Am 2001;32(1):135–70.
11. Abidi NA, Dhawan S, Gruen GS, et al. Wound-healing risk factors after open reduction and internal fixation of calcaneal fractures. Foot Ankle Int 1998; 19(12):856–61.
12. Shuler FD, Conti SF, Gruen GS, et al. Wound-healing risk factors after open reduction and internal fixation of calcaneal fractures: does correction of Bohler's angle alter outcomes? Orthop Clin North Am 2001;32(1):187–92.
13. Heier KA, Infante AF, Walling AK, et al. Open fractures of the calcaneus: soft-tissue injury determines outcome. J Bone Joint Surg Am 2003;85(12):2276–82.
14. Benirschke SK, Kramer PA. Wound healing complications in closed and open calcaneal fractures. J Orthop Trauma 2004;18(1):1–6.

15. Attinger C, Boehmler J. The foot and ankle reconstruction. In: Grabb and Smith's plastic Surgery. 6th edition. Lippincott Williams & Wilkins; 2007. p. 666–707.
16. Aldridge JM 3rd, Easley M, Nunley JA. Open calcaneal fractures: results of operative treatment. J Orthop Trauma 2004;18(1):7–11.
17. Thornton SJ, Cheleuitte D, Ptaszek AJ, et al. Treatment of open intra-articular calcaneal fractures: evaluation of a treatment protocol based on wound location and size. Foot Ankle Int 2006;27(5):317–23.
18. Canale ST. Campbell's operative orthopaedics. 10th edition. Philadelphia (PA): Mosby, Inc; 2003.
19. Buckwalter JA, Einhorn TA, Simon SR. Orthopaedic basic science- biology and biomechanics of the musculoskeletal system. 2nd edition. Philadelphia (PA): AAOS; 2000.
20. Palestro CJ, Caprioli R, Love C, et al. Rapid diagnosis of pedal osteomyelitis in diabetics with a technetium-99m-labeled monoclonal antigranulocyte antibody. J Foot Ankle Surg 2003;42(1):2–8.
21. Maskill JD, Bohay DR, Anderson JG. Calcaneus fractures: a review article. Foot Ankle Clin 2005;10(3):463–89.
22. Sanders R. Current concepts review – displaced intra-articular fractures of the calcaneus. J Bone Joint Surg Am 2000;82:225–50.
23. Herscovici D, Sanders RW, Scaduto JM, et al. Vacuum-assisted wound closure (VAC therapy) for the management of patients with high-energy soft tissue injuries. J Orthop Trauma 2003;17:683.
24. Saxena V, Hwang CW, Huang S, et al. Vacuum-assisted closure: microdeformations of wounds and cell proliferation. Plast Reconstr Surg 2004;114(5): 1086–96 [discussion: 1097–8].
25. Argenta LC, Morykwas MJ, Marks MW, et al. Vacuum-assisted closure: state of clinic art. Plast Reconstr Surg 2006;117(7 Suppl):127S–142S.
26. Beardmore AA, Brooks DE, Wenke JC, et al. Effectiveness of local antibiotic delivery with an osteoinductive and osteoconductive bone-graft substitute. J Bone Joint Surg Am 2005;87(1):107–12.
27. Chen SL, Chen TM, Chou TD, et al. Distally based sural fasciomusculocutaneous flap for chronic calcaneal osteomyelitis in diabetic patients. Ann Plast Surg 2005; 54(1):44–8.
28. del Pinal F, Herrero F, Cruz A. A technique to preserve the shape of the calcaneus after massive osteomyelitis. Br J Plast Surg 1999;52(5):415–7.
29. Yildirim S, Gideroglu K, Akoz T. The simple and effective choice for treatment of chronic calcaneal osteomyelitis: neurocutaneous flaps. Plast Reconstr Surg 2003; 111(2):753–60 [discussion: 761–2].
30. Levin LS. Foot and ankle soft-tissue deficiencies: who needs a flap? Am J Orthop 2006;35(1):11–9.
31. Baumhauer JF, Fraga CJ, Gould JS, et al. Total calcanectomy for the treatment of chronic calcaneal osteomyelitis. Foot Ankle Int 1998;19(12):849–55.
32. Smith DG. Principles of partial foot amputation in the diabetic. Foot Ankle 1997;2: 171 (Ptaszek ref).
33. Weinfeld SB, Schon LC. Amputations of the perimeters of the foot. Foot Ankle 1999;4:17 (Ptaszek ref).
34. Schwabegger AH, Shafighi M, Gurunluoglu R. Versatility of the abductor hallucis muscle as a conjoined or distally-based flap. J Trauma 2005;59(4):1007–11.

Syme's Ankle Disarticulation

Michael S. Pinzur, MD

KEYWORDS

• Syme ankle disarticulation • Diabetic dysvascular
• Traumatic injury • Transtibial amputation

In 1843, James Syme[1] listed three advantages for his technique of ankle disarticulation as compared with amputation at the transtibial level. He suggested that his operation would be less risky to patients than transtibial amputation and provide a more comfortable and functional amputation stump. Although current evidence supports his observations, this function and disability-sparing amputation level has not gained wide acceptance. This article addresses the demonstrated benefits associated with the Syme ankle disarticulation, provides clinical guidance for selecting appropriate patients, describes the surgery, and discusses avoiding and dealing with complications.

The foot is a uniquely adapted terminal end organ of weight bearing. The bony configuration allows the foot to be prepositioned in an unlocked position at heel strike, allowing the foot to function as a shock absorber. Advancing from heel strike through stance phase of gait, the foot rotates into a position of pronation, locking those same joints to create a stable starting block at push-off. This ability to preposition in various degrees of flexion-extension and pronation-supination gives the ability to adapt to uneven walking surfaces. This terminal weight-bearing organ is covered with durable protective plantar skin, which is capable of tolerating the application of high focal pressure and shearing forces. The intervening fibrous tissue of the heel pad and forefoot contain specially adapted fibrous septae capable of absorbing and transmitting the engineering loads of weight bearing to the bones of the foot. This highly efficient "machine" is driven by a coordinated interaction between the intrinsic and extrinsic musculature of the foot and ankle flexor and extensor muscles.[2] When these specially adapted tissues are lost, the loads associated with weight bearing must be absorbed by a single bony surface area that has little ability to dissipate and distribute these forces or adapt to uneven walking surfaces. It is the inability to adapt to changing loads and positions that leads to amputation stump pain or localized soft tissue breakdown.

Department of Orthopaedic Surgery and Rehabilitation, Loyola University Medical Center, 2160 South First Avenue, Maywood, IL 60153, USA
E-mail address: mpinzu1@lumc.edu

Foot Ankle Clin N Am 15 (2010) 487–494
doi:10.1016/j.fcl.2010.04.001
1083-7515/10/$ – see front matter © 2010 Elsevier Inc. All rights reserved.

FUNCTIONAL ADVANTAGES

The benefits associated with Syme ankle disarticulation can be divided into prosthetic weight bearing, mechanical efficiency, and energy cost of walking. The prosthetic advantage of the Syme ankle disarticulation, as compared with transtibial amputation, is the ability to directly bear weight on the normal retained heel pad. Direct load transfer (ie, end bearing within the prosthesis) allows the prosthetic socket simply to function in suspension. This is in contradistinction to the transtibial amputation stump that bears weight by indirect load transfer (ie, total surface bearing). Volume changes in the transtibial amputation stump lead to end bearing and tissue breakdown with volume loss and inability to don the prosthesis with volume gain.[3] Although not proved in the laboratory, many experts feel that end bearing also provides improved proprioception and stability during gait. Additionally, most experts suggest that a durable normal heel pad avoids stump ulcers more readily than the traditional transtibial amputation stump.

The second benefit is the ability to take advantage of a dynamic elastic response (so-called energy-storing) prosthetic foot. Partial foot amputees have a short lever arm capable of providing stability at terminal stance for push-off. Syme ankle disarticulation patients recover a relatively normal lever arm at push-off when using a prosthetic foot.[4] This ability to recover mechanical stability and a normal lever arm for propulsion explains the third advantage, a minimally increased metabolic cost of walking, compared with normal controls or partial foot amputees.[5–7]

PERIOPERATIVE ADVANTAGES

In patients with general anesthetic risk factors, the surgery can be performed with regional (ankle block) anesthesia and a calf tourniquet. Blood loss is decreased compared with transtibial or more proximal level amputation surgery. Patients require minimal postoperative prosthetic gait training and rarely require hospitalization in a rehabilitation unit. There is some retrospective uncontrolled data that suggest that diabetic and dysvascular patients survive longer after Syme amputation than similar patients undergoing transtibial amputation.[8,9]

INDICATIONS/CONTRAINDICIATIONS

Amputation should be performed as a preferred alternative to limb salvage when amputation has the probability to provide a better functional outcome. Prospective Syme amputees should have the rehabilitation potential to walk with a prosthesis after successful surgery. The heel pad should be clinically viable with normal tissue turgor. Local infection must be resolved before definitive wound closure. If a diabetic foot infection tracks into one of the 4 leg compartments, a thorough débridement and resolution of that infection should be accomplished before attempting Syme ankle disarticulation.

Patients should have adequate vascular inflow, as measured by palpable dorsalis pedis or posterior tibial pulses, ultrasound Doppler ankle-brachial index of 0.5 or better, or a transcutaneous partial pressure of oxygen ($TcPo_2$) of between 20 and 30 mm Hg.

In diabetic renal failure or polytrauma, patients are frequently malnourished after the resolution of a diabetic foot abscess or after a period of negative nitrogen balance after injury. If a patient's serum albumin level is below 2.5 g/dL, open wound management should be combined with culture-specific antibiotic therapy and nutritional support for a period of 1 to 2 weeks. Diabetic individuals without renal failure and normal trauma patients are able to recover wound healing potential. Their level of serum albumin demonstrates a significant rise within 7 to 10 days after control of systemic infection. Renal failure patients are unlikely to demonstrate a similar response. If they are incapable of raising their serum albumin level above 2.5 g/dL, more proximal amputation should be performed.

PREOPERATIVE PLANNING

The two most common applications of ankle disarticulation are nonreconstructable diabetic foot infection and trauma. Resolution of infection must be accomplished before definitive amputation wound closure. Débridement of all infected or nonviable tissue in the foot or involved leg compartments must be performed before wound closure. Infection-inducing malnutrition must also be reversed. There is no functional benefit that justifies the risk of wound failure in patients who do not have reasonable potential for successful prosthetic limb use.

Wound healing parameters for predicting successful amputation wound healing include vascular inflow, tissue nutrition, and immunocompentence. The minimum threshold arterial inflow capable of supporting wound healing is determined by an ultrasound Doppler ischemic ankle-brachial index of 0.5 or a $TcPo_2$ of between 20 and 30 mm Hg.[3,8,10–13] Transcutaneous oxygen tension should be measured after local tissue infection has been resolved, because $TcPo_2$ values can be falsely depressed in the presence of soft tissue infection.[14] It is generally accepted that amputation wound healing in diabetic patients requires minimum threshold levels of tissue nutrition (serum albumin of 3.0 g/dL) and immunocompetence (total lymphocyte count of 1500).[10–13,15–17] More recently, it has been observed that an amputation wound healing rate of 88% can be achieved after resolution of infection once the serum albumin reaches a level of 2.5 g/dL.[8] It also seems that total lymphocyte count may not be as valid a predictor of wound healing.

TECHNIQUE

Wagner[15,16] originally performed the procedure in 2 stages, as a method to avoid infection. The surgery can achieve similar success rates when performed in a single stage.[10] A fishmouth incision is used with the apices of the flaps located at the anterior midpoints of the medial and lateral malleoli (**Fig. 1**). This differs slightly from Wagner's recommended incision, where the apices are located at a point 1 to 1.5 cm anterior and distal to the tips of the medial and lateral malleoli. Moving the apices proximal and posterior minimizes the large medial and lateral dog-ears that were removed at the time of Wagner's second-stage operation when he removed the malleoli.

The incision is carried sharply to bone, where the calcaneus and talus are removed using sharp dissection (**Fig. 2**). Care should be taken to protect the posterior tibialis artery, which is the primary source of blood supply to the distal flap. Traction is applied to the talus with a bone hook or bone-holding clamp to facilitate the sharp dissection necessary to accomplish the bony resection while avoiding traumatic injury to the remaining heel pad. Care should be taken to avoid puncturing the poorly padded skin overlying the insertion of the Achilles tendon. Historically, it has been taught that puncturing the skin at this point dooms the healing of the flap. Although a drainage hole at this point in the surgery is best avoided, survival or failure of the flap is more dependant on the gentle handling of the tissues and preservation of the posterior tibial arterial blood supply.[8,10]

Once the ankle is disarticulated, the medial and lateral malleoli are removed flush with the articular surface of the distal tibia, retaining the resilient weight-bearing

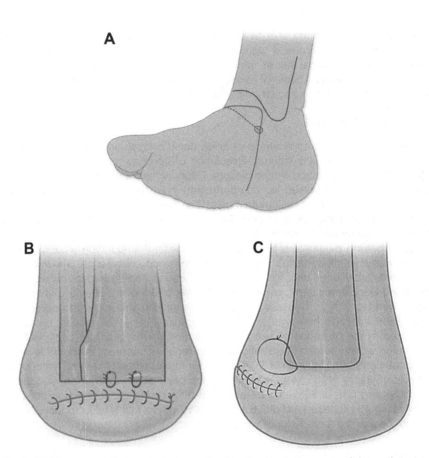

Fig. 1. (*A*) The current 1-stage technique of ankle disarticulation uses a fishmouth incision with the apices at the anterior midpoints of the medial and lateral malleoli, shown in the figure as a solid line. This differs from Wagner's 2-stage technique (*dotted line*) in which the apices are located at a point 1 to 1.5 cm distal and anterior to the tips of the medial and lateral malleoli. (*B*) After disarticulation of the ankle, the malleoli are removed flush with the articular surface of the distal tibia, preserving the articular cartilage of the distal tibia for weight bearing. The flares of the medial and lateral malleoli are removed in line with the diaphysis of the tibia and fibula. This narrows the otherwise bulbous amputation stump and provides a raw bony surface adding stability to the heel pad. (*C*) Oblique drill holes are made in the anterior distal tibia. The heel pad is secured to the tibia via these drill holes, using nonabsorbable suture. (*Reprinted from* Pinzur MS, Stuck R, Sage R, et al. Syme's ankle disarticulation in patients with diabetes. J Bone Joint Surg 2003;85A:1667–72; with permission.)

articular cartilage of the tibia. The metaphyseal flares of the malleoli are removed flush with the corresponding diaphysis of the respective tibia and fibula. Removing the malleoli in this fashion creates a more narrow and cosmetic residual limb, avoiding the bulbous, wide ankle that had previously been unsightly to patients.

Migration of the heel pad has historically compromised functional prosthetic fitting. This can be prevented by two surgical steps taken before wound closure. Removing the metaphyseal flares of the distal tibia and fibula creates areas of exposed metaphyseal bone. The medial and lateral soft tissue envelope tends to adhere to the exposed

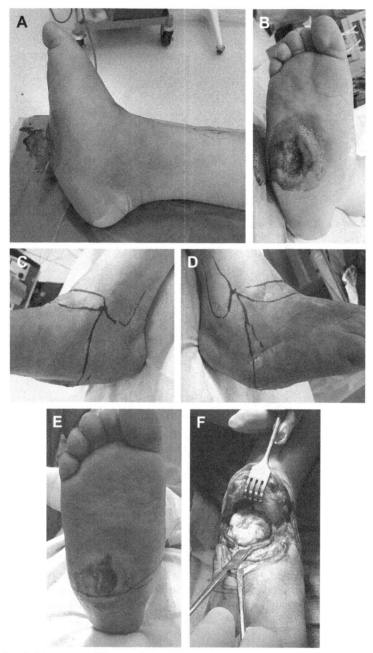

Fig. 2. (*A, B*) This 36-year-old type I diabetic had a failed attempt at reconstruction for Charcot foot arthropathy. She had persistent draining osteomyelitis and was not willing to undergo another attempt at limb reconstruction. (*C, D*) Surgical incision. (*E*) Note that the plantar flap length dictated making the incision just proximal to the open plantar wound. (*F*) The incision is made directly down to bone. The ankle joint is entered anteriorly and sharp dissection is used to excise the talus and calcaneus. A bone clamp or bone hook is used to pull the talus and calcaneus forward to facilitate sharp dissection and protection of the posterior skin and the plantar keel pad. (*G*) The lateral and medial malleoli are removed flush with the retained articular surface of the tibia. The metaphyseal flares of the malleoli are removed flush with the outer borders of the two bones. (*H*) Two or three drill holes are made in the anterior corner of the tibia. The heel pad is secured to the tibia via these drill holes. (*I*) The dog-ears will remodel over time.

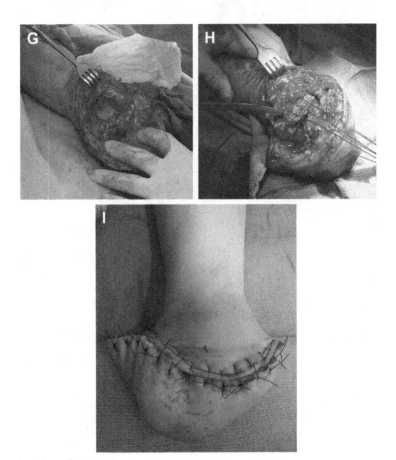

Fig. 2. (*continued*)

metaphyseal bone, if the heel pad is secured to the distal tibia via drill holes. Two or three oblique drill holes can be made in the distal anterior tibia for securing the heel pad with stout nonabsorbable sutures. Smith and colleagues[18] secure the heel pad by attaching the detached Achilles tendon to the posterior distal surface of the tibia before wound closure. Suction drains for the first 24 hours are optional. The deep tissues are reapproximated with one layer of heavy absorbable sutures. The skin can be repaired with sutures or skin staples.

COMPLICATIONS

The wound-healing rate of this amputation level is slightly lower than the expected 90% rate in other diabetic lower-extremity amputations. Many of the wounds have areas of delayed healing that eventually heal by secondary intention.[19] Heal pad migration can generally be avoided by one of the methods described previously. Delayed wound healing or superficial wound infections can be managed with local wound care. Deep infection, especially when the anchoring suture is involved, requires débridement and removal of the anchoring suture. After resolution of the infection, the anchoring sutures need to be reattached at the time of secondary wound closure.

POSTOPERATIVE MANAGEMENT

Suction drains are optional, based on the experience of the operating surgeon. A rigid plaster dressing is advised at the time of the first dressing change to protect the wound from external trauma or falls during transfer or ambulation. A new total contact cast with a rubber walking heel can be applied as early as 7 to 10 days after surgery to allow weight bearing. A volume adaptable preparatory prosthesis can be used in the early postoperative period until the residual limb volume and shape stabilize.

DISCUSSION

Like knee disarticulation, most orthopedic surgeons avoid Syme amputation as a treatment option because they were not exposed to the technique during their residency. When the guidelines described in this article are applied, reasonable success rates can be achieved. Compared with transtibial amputation in similar patients, rehabilitation is far less complex. Patients rarely require hospitalization in a rehabilitation unit and rarely require more than minimal physical therapy gait training.

It has been retrospectively observed that diabetic dysvascular patients seem to achieve greater walking independence and survive longer than similar patients undergoing transtibial amputation.[8] It is unknown whether or not this is a real effect of the surgery or if patients undergoing Syme amputation have less severe vascular and cardiac disease.

Experts agree that traumatic Syme amputees are less functionally impaired than traumatic transtibial amputees.[20] It might also be argued that traumatic Syme amputees are less impaired than a partial foot amputees. This argument can be made because of the retention of a normal lever arm at push-off with a Syme amputation and prosthesis as opposed to a partial foot amputee with a shortened lever arm.[4] It might be argued that this lever arm could be achieved if partial foot amputees used an ankle foot orthosis combined with a prosthetic shoe filler. Unfortunately, it has been observed that most partial foot amputees reject the encumbrance of such a device.

Whichever perspective is taken, it is apparent that the Syme ankle disarticulation is underused in American medicine. Once the learning curve is overcome, improved functional outcomes can be offered to few diabetic dysvascular and traumatic injured patients.

REFERENCES

1. Syme J. Amputation at the ankle joint. Lond edinburg monthly. J Med Sci 1843; 2:93.
2. Mann RA. In: Coughlin MJ, Mann RA, editors. Surgery of the foot and ankle. 7th edition. St. Louis (MO): Mosby; 1999. p. 2–35.
3. Pinzur MS. New concepts in lower-limb amputation and prosthetic management. Instr Course Lect 1990;39:361–6.
4. Pinzur MS, Wolf B, Havey RM. Walking pattern of midfoot and ankle disarticulation amputees. Foot Ankle Int 1997;18:635–8.
5. Pinzur MS, Gold J, Schwartz D, et al. Energy demands for walking in dysvascular amputees as related to the level of amputation. Orthopedics 1992;15:1033–7.
6. Fisher SV, Gullickson G. Energy cost of ambulation in health and disability: a literature review. Arch Phys Med Rehabil 1978;59:124–33.
7. Waters RL, Perry J, Antonelli D, et al. Energy cost of walking of amputees: the influence of level of amputation. J Bone Joint Surg Am 1976;58:42–6.

8. Pinzur MS, Stuck R, Sage R, et al. Syme's ankle disarticulation in patients with diabetes. J Bone Joint Surg Am 2003;85:1667–72.

9. Pinzur MS, Gottschalk F, Smith D, et al. Functional outcome of below-knee amputation in peripheral vascular insufficiency. Clin Orthop 1993;286:247–9.

10. Pinzur MS, Smith DG, Osterman H. Syme ankle disarticulation in peripheral vascular disease and diabetic foot infection: the one-stage versus two-stage procedure. Foot Ankle Int 1995;16:124–7.

11. Pinzur MS, Sage R, Stuck R, et al. Transcutaneous oxygen as a predictor of wound healing in amputations of the foot and ankle. Foot Ankle 1992;13:271–2.

12. Pinzur M, Morrison C, Sage R, et al. Syme's two-stage amputation in insulin-requiring diabetics with gangrene of the forefoot. Foot Ankle 1991;11:394–6.

13. Dickhaut SC, DeLee JC, Page CP. Nutritional status: importance in predicting wound healing after amputation. J Bone Joint Surg Am 1984;66:71–5.

14. Pinzur MS, Stuck R, Sage R, et al. Transcutaneous oxygen tension in the dysvascular foot with infection. Foot Ankle 1993;14:254–6.

15. Wagner FW Jr. Management of the diabetic neurotrophic foot. Part II. A classification and treatment program for diabetic, neuropathic, and dysvascular foot problems. In: Instructional course lectures, the American Academy of Orthopaedic Surgeons, 28. St. Louis (MO): C.V. Mosby; 1979. p. 143–65.

16. Wagner FW Jr. Amputations of the foot and ankle. Current status. Clin Orthop 1977;122:62–9.

17. Pinzur MS, Kaminsky M, Sage R, et al. Amputations at the middle level of the foot. J Bone Joint Surg Am 1986;68:1061–4.

18. Smith DG, Sangeorzan BJ, Hansen ST, et al. Achilles tendon tenodesis to prevent heel pad migration in the Syme's amputation. Foot Ankle 1994;15:14–7.

19. Smith DG, Berke GM. Post-operative management of the lower extremity amputee. J Prosthet Orthot 2004;16(Suppl):3.

20. Miller LA, McCay JA. Summary and conclusions from the Academy's Sixth State-of-the-Science Conference on lower limb prosthetic outcomes measures. Hagerstown (MD): Lippincott Williams and Wilkins; 2006. American Academy of Orthotists and Prosthetists.

Risk and Prevention of Reulceration After Partial Foot Amputation

Ronald A. Sage, DPM[a,b,*]

KEYWORDS

• Diabetic ulcers • Foot amputation • Callus • Foot pressures

Partial foot amputations account for half of more than 80,000 amputations per year related to diabetes in the United States. Many of these amputations result from minor repetitive trauma associated with chronic pressure points and callus formation in the foot. Changes in weight-bearing patterns after partial foot amputations frequently lead to new focal pressure points and keratosis, resulting in subsequent ulceration in neuropathic and dysvascular patients. The minor trauma, ulceration, and faulty wound healing associated with these pressure points are frequent contributing factors to further amputation. Prevention of reulceration starts with medical management of the macrovascular and microvascular complications of diabetes. Beyond that, if a new focal pressure point is identified after partial foot amputation, prescription of an appropriate pressure-relieving orthosis or prosthesis may reduce the risk of reulceration. The risk of reulceration may also be reduced when shoes and orthotic prescriptions are combined with foot evaluation and management services as necessary to control focal callus formation before ulceration can occur. Simple paring of thick keratotic lesions at appropriate intervals is effective in reducing focal pressure and associated risk of ulceration. The partially amputated foot must be considered at high risk for further ulceration and amputation and requires careful follow-up long after the surgical site is healed.

AMPUTATIONS AND THE DIABETIC FOOT

The number of amputations performed in the United States because of diabetes continues to rise, in spite of efforts to control diabetes and improve limb salvage rates. More than 80,000 amputations are performed each year, with approximately one half of them transtibial or higher and one half partial foot procedures.[1] Partial foot

[a] Section of Podiatry, Department of Orthopaedic Surgery and Rehabilitation, Loyola University Chicago, Stritch School of Medicine, 2160 South First Avenue, Maywood, IL 60153, USA
[b] Edward Hines Jr VA Hospital, Hines, IL 60141, USA
* Section of Podiatry, Department of Orthopaedic Surgery and Rehabilitation, Loyola University Stritch School of Medicine, 2160 South First Avenue, Maywood, IL 60153.
E-mail address: rsage@lumc.edu

Foot Ankle Clin N Am 15 (2010) 495–500
doi:10.1016/j.fcl.2010.04.006
1083-7515/10/$ – see front matter © 2010 Published by Elsevier Inc.

foot.theclinics.com

amputations are performed to preserve most of the lower extremity affected by limb-threatening infection or ischemia. Limb-threatening conditions include severe ulcerations, osteomyelitis, and gangrene secondary to vascular disease. The procedures performed to treat these conditions include toe amputation, ray resection, and transmetatarsal, Lisfranc, Chopart, and Syme amputations. Successful wound healing of these procedures depends on adequate vascular perfusion, which is frequently present in neuropathic feet, but may require endovascular or bypass procedures in dysvascular extremities. Once healed, partial foot amputations are at risk for reulceration and further amputation. With careful long-term postoperative management, however, preventive interventions may be initiated that can reduce the risk of further amputation and preserve the remaining extremity salvaged by a partial foot amputation.

Many complications can occur after virtually any partial foot amputation, leading to deformities they may suffer further ulcerations. Toe amputations can lead to contractures or hammering of adjacent toes. Second toe amputations can lead to hallux valgus. Ray resections performed for ulceration and infection of a metatarsal head can develop transfer ulcerations of the adjacent metatarsal head. Midfoot amputations, especially those at the Lisfranc or Chopart level, can develop equinus. All of these procedures should be monitored well after healing is achieved to observe for preulcerative pressure points requiring further management.

COMPLICATIONS OF DIABETES

Pecoraro and colleagues[2] described three causal pathways that lead to amputation in the diabetic foot: minor trauma, cutaneous ulceration, and faulty wound healing. Diabetic patients suffer from macrovascular and microvascular complications contributing to faulty wound healing. Prevention of further amputation requires medical management of the factors leading to these complications. Surgeons should encourage their patients' compliance with measures to manage these disease processes, which include glucose control, blood pressure control, lipid management, diet, and exercise.[3]

Macrovascular complications affect the larger vessels and include coronary artery disease (CAD) and peripheral artery disease (PAD). Although diabetics are thought to be more susceptible to these conditions than the nondiabetic population, glucose control alone does not alter the course of these diseases. Medical interventions include exercise, prevention of thrombosis with aspirin or other medications, control of hypertension, and lipid management.

Hypertension education and compliance with blood pressure control measures need to be encouraged. Undiagnosed or uncontrolled high blood pressure should be referred to a primary physician for intervention. Screening for PAD by Doppler examination and determination of ankle-brachial artery index can provide an indication of vascular disease and can also aid the detection of CAD. Patients over 50 years old with an ankle-brachial artery index less than 0.5 should have cardiovascular risk evaluation. There is a 20% 5-year risk of nonfatal cardiac events in patients diagnosed with PAD and a 30% 5-year mortality rate in this group, even if they have not suffered from critical limb ischemia or amputation.[4] Medical interventions can include thrombosis risk prevention, exercise, and management of lipid abnormalities. Referral for vascular intervention is appropriate when the ankle-brachial artery index is abnormal, especially in cases of claudication or tissue loss.

Microvascular complications include retinopathy, renal disease, and neuropathy. These seem to be directly related to hyperglycemia. Optimizing glucose monitoring and control is the standard of care for type 1 and type 2 diabetic mellitus. Encouraging compliance with such a regimen should be part of the postoperative follow-up. Severe signs of neuropathy, such as profound numbness or ulceration, are indicators of poor control. Office evaluation of blood glucose or hemoglobin A1c may provide laboratory evidence of poor control. Patients should be encouraged to monitor and report their glucose levels to the physician caring for their diabetes and obtain appropriate management to optimize their blood glucose levels. Referral to an endocrinologist may be helpful if the primary physician is unable to normalize the glucose levels.

FOOT RISK IDENTIFICATION

The American Diabetes Association, in a position statement on foot care, has identified four conditions that are associated with an increased risk of amputation.[5] These include:

Peripheral neuropathy
Altered biomechanics
   Pressure callus
   Limited joint mobility, bony deformity, or severe nail pathology
Peripheral vascular disease
History of ulcer or amputation.

Partial foot amputees are almost by definition affected by most, if not all, of these risk factors. In particular, minor trauma associated with pressure points or focal pressure callus frequently leads to ulcerations that fail to heal in neuropathic patients.[6,7] A focal pressure keratosis is a well-defined area of thickening of the keratin layer of the skin occurring in response to intermittent localized pressure. These can appear plantarly under any metatarsal head or bony prominence as calluses. They can appear dorsally over phalangeal heads as corns or over bunions at the first or fifth metatarsal heads. In nondiabetic, sensate patients, these corns and calluses are painful and may prompt patients to rest, alter their footgear, or seek treatment. In neuropathic diabetic patients, they are painless, and there is little or no motivation to rest, protect, or treat the keratosis. Eventually, the worsening callus develops blistering, hemorrhage, and ulceration. If a partial foot amputation has been performed because of a nonhealing focal pressure ulceration, there is a significant risk of the altered biomechanics after surgery, leading to a transfer of the focal pressure point to another location in the residual foot, starting the ulcerative process all over again. These patients can have even more problems healing if PAD is also present and not treated. The new keratosis is unlikely to show up until well after patients have healed the surgical procedure. It will only occur after patients resume near-normal ambulation and, because of neuropathy, is likely to be painless. Identification and management of new keratotic lesions before they can ulcerate requires follow-up visits on regular intervals by a surgeon or a provider interested in treating these problems before they require further operations **Fig. 1**.

Among the measures to be taken if new focal pressure points occur are prescription of a pressure-relieving foot orthosis and accommodative footgear. At times a simple athletic shoe or inlay depth shoe with a commercial insole may be adequate to control the pressure point. Alternatively, some patients with severe hemorrhagic keratosis under an isolated bony prominence may require custom orthotics, ankle-foot orthoses, or even charcot restraint orthotic walkers in addition to débridement of the keratosis on a regular basis to prevent ulceration. The application of these fundamental orthotic and podiatric principles is extremely effective in preventing ulceration,

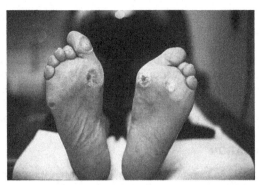

Fig. 1. At-risk feet with focal pressure calluses. Note the patient's left foot with residual callus after amputation of second toe.

infection, hospitalization, and amputation. This care is provided and these devices are prescribed and fabricated on the basis of experience and consensus, however, and hard evidence is lacking to support their appropriate use.

OUTPATIENT CARE AND MORBIDITY REDUCTION

In 2001, the author's group at Loyola University Chicago and Edward Hines Jr VA Hospital reviewed 233 cases of diabetic foot ulceration admitted to those hospitals over a 7-year period and found that 82% of these ulcers were preceded by a focal pressure keratosis. Those patients who had frequent outpatient clinic care had significantly lower-grade ulcerations and were significantly less likely to require any form of surgical intervention. Conversely, the worst ulcerations were in those without documentation of any prior foot care. Measures that were found effective in decreasing ulcer grade included débridement of keratosis or ulcer, prescription of protective shoes, and patient education.[8]

The clinic visits consisted of identification of patient complaints and pertinent history. Foot complaints and comorbidities, such as renal disease or CAD, were documented, medications reviewed, and assessment of glucose control noted. The visits included a brief vascular and sensory evaluation. Detailed examination of these systems was not considered necessary at every visit but should be performed once or twice a year depending on individual patients. In particular, the presence or absence of ulcer or preulcerative keratosis was noted. Diagnosis and risk assessment were stated. The patients were educated about these findings and instructed in appropriate home care and self-examination. They were advised to seek urgent attention should evidence of blistering, drainage, color change, or ulceration occur. Calluses were pared, ulcerative lesions débrided, and protective shoes and orthotics prescribed as necessary.

Management of focal pressure keratosis, when present, is essential to lower the risk of further ulceration. Such management includes prescription for pressure-relieving shoes and orthoses. Existing footgear should be inspected and replacement or revision prescribed when necessary. Débridement of chronic pressure keratosis at intervals appropriate to prevent ulceration can decrease infections, hospitalizations, and amputations. These intervals are based on frequent follow-up visits. Depending on the thickness or signs of blistering and hemorrhagic discoloration, visits may be necessary every 2 to 3 months or, in some cases, as frequently as every 2 to 3 weeks.

The natural history of an untreated pressure callus in diabetic neuropathic patients is ulceration, infection, and amputation. Patients should be educated, about the risk of complications from pressure callus. Clinicians should be attentive to the need to manage pressure callus before this chain of events can occur. The minor trauma associated with focal pressure callus leading to ulceration, faulty healing, infection, and amputation is a classic example of Pecoraro's triad, which Pecoraro and colleagues stated is responsible for 80% of all diabetes-related amputations.[2]

Patient education should be provided at every follow-up. Neuropathy and the importance of visual foot examinations at home can be explained. Good skin care and hygiene principles can be reviewed. Compliance with diabetes control and cardiovascular risk reduction measures should be encouraged. Indications for professional treatment should be explained. Appropriate intervals for office visits should be determined and recommended. Patients should be advised to seek urgent attention for any significant change in the appearance of their feet or any, even minor, injury.

SUMMARY

Altered biomechanics of the foot can lead to focal pressure keratosis. In diabetic patients, this is an event that can initiate the triad of minor trauma, cutaneous ulceration, and faulty healing thought to lead to most diabetes-related amputations. This is especially true in poorly controlled diabetics or in those patients with vascular disease. Partial foot amputation alters the biomechanics of weight bearing making patients susceptible to new pressure points that can ulcerate.

Orthotic and prosthetic care after partial foot amputation differs in diabetic patients, who have many medical issues and are at risk for further amputation, from posttraumatic amputees who seek optimum function and performance from their prosthetics and orthotics. The ideal foot orthotic or prosthetic in diabetic patients at risk for further amputation must disperse, cushion, or prevent focal pressure points. To improve on such devices, research needs to be directed at identifying the likely points of maximum pressure after various partial foot amputations. Devices and materials need to be studied to determine how an orthosis or prosthesis can effectively eliminate or redirect these pressure points and reduce the risk of reulceration. Paring of keratotic lesions also decreases focal pressure and can present ulceration if performed at appropriate intervals. Reducing focal pressure in the partially amputated diabetic foot reduces the likelihood of subsequent amputation and requires careful clinical follow-up of the at risk foot.

REFERENCES

1. Reiber GE. Epidemiology and health care costs of diabetic foot problems. In: Veves A, Giurini JM, LoGerfo FW, editors. The diabetic foot: medical and surgical management. Totowa (NJ): Humana Press; 2002. p. 39–50.
2. Pecoraro RE, Reiber GE, Burgess EM. Pathways to diabetic limb amputation: basis for prevention. Diabetes Care 1990;13:513–21.
3. Sheehan P. Introduction to diabetes. In: Veves A, Giurini JM, LoGerfo FW, editors. The diabetic foot: medical and surgical management. Totowa (NJ): Humana Press; 2002. p. 1–34.
4. American Diabetes Association Consensus Statement. Peripheral arterial disease in people with diabetes. Diabetes Care 2003;26:3333–41.
5. Mayfield JA, Reiber GE, Sanders LJ, et al. Preventive foot care in people with diabetes, technical review and position statement. Diabetes Care 1998;21:2161–79.

6. Lyons TE, Rich J, Veves A. Foot pressure abnormalities in the diabetic foot. In: Veves A, Giurini JM, LoGerfo FW, editors. The diabetic foot: medical and surgical management. Totowa (NJ): Humana Press; 2002. p. 127–46.

7. VanSchie CHM, Boulton AJM. Biomechanics of the diabetic foot: the road to ulceration. In: Veves A, Giurini JM, LoGerfo FW, editors. The diabetic foot: medical and surgical management. Totowa (NJ): Humana Press; 2002. p. 147–58.

8. Sage RA, Webster JK, Fisher SG. Out patient care and morbidity reduction in diabetic foot ulcers associated with chronic pressure callous. J Am Podiatr Med Assoc 2001;91:275–91.

Gait Abnormality Following Amputation in Diabetic Patients

Richard M. Marks, MD[a],*, Jason T. Long, PhD[a,b],
Emily L. Exten, MD[a]

KEYWORDS

- Center of pressure • Transmetatarsal amputation
- Ground reaction force • Extensor hallucis brevis

Amputations of the lower extremity may result from several etiologic factors. Most amputations performed in the United States result from a dysvascular limb. A majority of the population with vascular impairment comprises people with diabetes. These individuals frequently have comorbidities that may also affect the ultimate outcome of amputation. Loss of protective sensation, propensity toward infection, and visual and balance impairment all create additional issues with postamputation gait in the population with diabetes.

Indications for amputation include the sequelae of trauma, vascular impairment, infection, dysfunctional limb, congenital malformations, and tumor resection. Trauma to the lower extremities may result in amputation, either from severe bone loss, soft tissue degloving, arterial compromise with dysvascular changes, or subsequent infection that is not amenable to limb salvage. Peripheral vascular disease, particularly when associated with diabetes mellitus, accounts for more than 150,000 amputations per year. As of 2005, 54% of amputees in the United States suffered dysvascular disease, and two-thirds of those patients were diabetic.[1] It has been estimated that diabetes and its comorbidities account for 50% of lower extremity amputations worldwide.

People with diabetes have a 20-fold higher amputation rate compared with the general population.[2] A review of 12-month reamputation and mortality rates by Dillingham and colleagues[3] revealed that 26% of amputees required additional amputation procedures, and that one-third died within 1 year of the index amputation. If the initial amputation level was at the foot level, the reamputation rate increased to 34%.

[a] Department of Orthopaedic Surgery, Medical College of Wisconsin, 9200 West Wisconsin Avenue, Milwaukee, WI 53226, USA
[b] Orthopaedic & Rehabilitation Engineering Center (OREC), Marquette University, Medical College of Wisconsin, WI, USA
* Corresponding author. Division of Foot & Ankle Surgery, Department of Orthopaedic Surgery, Medical College of Wisconsin, 9200 West Wisconsin Avenue, Milwaukee, WI 53226.
E-mail address: RMarks@mcw.edu

Foot Ankle Clin N Am 15 (2010) 501–507
doi:10.1016/j.fcl.2010.05.001
1083-7515/10/$ – see front matter © 2010 Elsevier Inc. All rights reserved.

Amputees who had diabetes were younger, more likely to be men, underwent their first amputation at an earlier age, died at an earlier age, and were more likely to require progression to a higher amputation level.

GAIT

Normal gait can be defined as the translation of the center of gravity through space in the manner that uses energy most efficiently.[4] Gait is subdivided into periods of weight-bearing and nonweight-bearing. The weight-bearing "stance" begins when the foot first contacts the ground "foot contact" and lasts until the foot leaves the ground ("foot-off"). The nonweight-bearing "swing" phase begins at foot-off and continues until the next foot contact. Together, stance and swing make up the unit of gait cycle normalization known as the "stride" (**Fig. 1**). In normal gait, the stance phase makes up 62% of the gait cycle and the swing phase makes up 38% of the cycle. Stance and swing can be further divided into biomechanically relevant subphases. Weight-bearing subphases include initial contact (0%–2% gait cycle), loading response (2%–10% cycle), midstance (10%–30% cycle), terminal stance (30%–50% cycle), and preswing (10%–62% cycle). Nonweight-bearing subphases include initial swing (62%–73% cycle), midswing (73%–87% cycle), and terminal swing (87%–100% cycle).

During initial contact and loading response, key angular modifications occur in the foot and ankle, which allow the lower extremity to accept loading while minimizing impact forces. Following foot contact, the tibia rotates internally, the subtalar joint pronates, and the transverse tarsal joint unlocks and shifts to a parallel orientation. These motions allow the gradual shift of weight from the posterolateral edge of the foot to the medial edge. During this process, impact forces are dissipated by the progressive flattening of the arches of the midfoot. During initial contact, eccentric activity of the tibialis anterior controls the descent of the toes to the floor.

Following loading response, activity ceases in the tibialis anterior. The midstance and terminal stance phases are marked by relative ankle dorsiflexion as the tibia progresses forward over the plantigrade foot. Concurrent eccentric activity is observed in the gastrocnemius muscle to control this forward progress. As weight shifts from the hindfoot to the forefoot, the body's center of pressure (CoP) moves distally and the foot acts as a lever arm. Contraction of the tibialis posterior leads to subtalar inversion, shifting the gastrocnemius muscle into a more medial position, which optimizes its ability as an ankle plantarflexor. Concurrent external tibia rotation is observed, and the transverse tarsal joint begins to engage and lock. As the CoP completes its distal translation, the rigid foot is used as a lever to transmit energy from the gastrocnemius to the lower extremity for push-off.

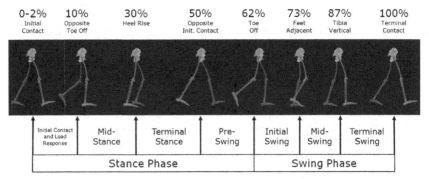

Fig. 1. Gait cycle events and phases.

Following push-off, the tibialis anterior activates to pull the toes up for floor clearance. Aside from this activity, the majority of the swing phase is passive, with rectus femoris and hamstring activity noted late in swing to decelerate the lower extremity and stabilize the hip in preparation for the next foot contact.

Gait difficulties in the population with diabetes are associated with the prevalence of sensory neuropathy, which can affect balance and proprioceptive capabilities. The walking performance of diabetic patients with neuropathy has been compared with diabetic patients with ulcers, transmetatarsal amputations (TMAs), and transtibial amputations.[5] Walking capacity and performance (gait count, stride count) decreased with the progression of foot complications. The maximum peak pressures of patients with foot ulcers and partial foot amputations were higher than those with diabetic neuropathy. On the contralateral foot, the ulcer group had higher peak pressures over the total foot, and patients with partial foot amputations and transtibial amputations had higher peak pressures over the heel.

AMPUTATION CONSIDERATIONS

The diabetic person with a lower extremity amputation faces not only inherent limitations from neuropathy, proprioceptive, and balance difficulties, but must also adjust to limitations imposed by the specific levels of amputation. In addition, the population with diabetes also has a higher incidence of heart disease, peripheral vascular disease, and retinopathy, which may affect the ability to ambulate at an effective pace and to consume energy. Prosthetic usage imposes increased energy demands from using the proximal musculature to substitute for the sacrificed distal musculature. Other factors affecting energy expenditure include the adequacy of the prosthetic fit, type of prosthesis,[6] and shoe modifications[7-9] as well as experience in using the prosthetic and shoe modifications. For those individuals that forgo a prosthesis, upper extremity weight-bearing demands also create additional energy demands. Several studies have evaluated the effect of amputation level on the oxygen (O_2) cost, which factors in velocity of gait and O_2 rate. The O_2 cost increases progressively as the amputation level becomes more proximal.[10-12] Patients with a transtibial (T-T) amputation have a 20% higher O_2 cost and less efficient gait compared with able-bodied subjects.[12-15] Vascular amputees, many of whom were diabetic, fared poorer than the traumatic amputees.[16]

Amputee gait is affected by a change in the length of the foot lever arm. Weight progression of the stance leg is altered or absent, resulting in loss of energy absorption and forward propulsion.[17] The shorter foot diminishes the ground contact and decreases the functional lever arm of the foot[10]; this creates faster weight transfer to the normal limb, leading to increased loads being absorbed on the normal limb. The residual limb also absorbs more of the ground reaction force (GRF), creating more stress on the residual limb and more energy demands with ambulation.[18]

FOREFOOT AMPUTATIONS

Amputations of the forefoot consist of toe, hallux, or ray resections. Single-toe amputations tend to be well tolerated; however, they may result in secondary deformities of adjacent digits. Walking speed does not tend to be affected; however, running and jumping activities may be compromised. Weight distribution over the affected foot or contralateral foot tends to be minimally changed.

Amputation of the hallux should take care to maintain the base of the proximal phalanx to preserve the insertion of the extensor hallucis brevis (EHB), plantar fascia, and sesamoids. Loss of these structures may result in weight transfer laterally and loss of push-off strength.[19] Amputation proximal to the metatarsophalangeal (MTP) joints has been shown to significantly diminish power generated across the ankle, with significant wasting of the triceps surae musculature.[20] The lack of ankle power generation results in adaptive gait, whereby the hip becomes the primary source of power to advance the body forward; this reflects the role of the ankle plantarflexors to accelerate the leg forward into swing phase and maintain the vertical height of the center of mass of the upper body. Once the level of amputation was proximal to the MTP joints, power loss was similar for transmetatarsal, Lisfranc, and Chopart amputations.[20] There was no advantage in preserving residual foot length once the MTP joints were sacrificed. Mann and colleagues[21] evaluated the gait of 10 patients who underwent pollicization of the hallux with amputation through the MTP joint. No difference was seen in cadence, step length, stance phase time, or swing phase time. No kinetic changes in the sagittal and transverse planes, or angular motion of the pelvis, hip femur, or tibia were noted. In the foot with the amputated toe, the line of progression of the CoP was located more laterally, with a decrease in the forward progression. Increased activity did tend to transfer stresses under the second and third metatarsal heads. Plantar aponeurosis and loss of the intrinsic muscular insertions results in loss of the windlass mechanism and elevation of the medial longitudinal arch. The destabilization of the first MTP joint decreases contact loading of the hallux and prevents the forward and medial progression of the CoP during weight bearing.

Ray resections may result in shifts of the weight-bearing pattern to the adjacent metatarsal heads.[22] Lateral-ray resections tend to be better tolerated. Care should be taken to preserve the metatarsal base. Loss of the base of the first metatarsal may destabilize the attachment of the peroneus longus or tibialis anterior, resulting in loss of plantarflexion of the medial column and ankle dorsiflexion. The base of the fifth metatarsal should be preserved to maintain the attachment of the peroneus brevis. Loss of this attachment may result in adduction of the forefoot and equinovarus.

TRANSMETATARSAL AMPUTATION

Many investigators prefer TMA to a more proximal amputation because it preserves ankle function, maintains a distal weight-bearing surface, and maintains a more energy-efficient gait.[23] With more proximal amputations, the dorsiflexors may be compromised, resulting in an equinus contracture. In some cases, lengthening of the tendo achilles may be necessary to prevent an equinus contracture. If the peroneus brevis attachment is compromised, equinovarus deformity may result. The shorter foot decreases ground contact and creates a shorter functional lever arm, resulting in increased stress on the residual limb and decreased ambulation efficiency. Significantly greater peak plantar pressures have been recorded in individuals with TMA as well as lower peak plantar pressures in the heels.[24] Greater maximum dynamic dorsiflexion range of motion is seen in intact feet as compared with the TMA. Loss of the functional length of the foot lever arm and a decreased ability of the posterior calf musculature to control forward motion of the tibia from midstance to toe-off is also observed.[25] Shoewear and insert modifications may reduce plantar pressures in diabetic patients with TMA.[26] A full-length shoe with total contact insert and rigid rockerbottom sole, or short shoe with rigid rockerbottom tends to be most effective in preventing ulceration and better distribution of contact pressures.[27]

MIDFOOT AMPUTATIONS

Lisfranc and Chopart amputations further shorten the residual lever arm, while increasing the risk of equinovarus deformity due to the unopposed force of the plantarflexors. Reattachment of the tibialis anterior and peroneus brevis can lessen this occurrence, and it may be necessary to concomitantly lengthen the tendo achilles. The Lisfranc amputation disarticulates the foot at the tarso-metatarsal junction, and is performed if bone or soft tissue compromise precludes TMA. Prosthetic modifications similar to those used for the TMA are used to decrease the force on the residual limb during terminal gait. A longer toe plate and rocker sole are designed to decrease GRFs on the terminal residual limb.[11,28]

Chopart amputation tends to be poorly tolerated by active individuals because of limitations with push-off and stability, but tends to be better tolerated by limited ambulators who require stability for functional transfers. Chopart amputation also maintains ankle motion and residual limb length.[29] Reattachment of the tibialis anterior helps prevent equinus deformity, and tendo achilles lengthening is helpful. Balance between the tibialis posterior and peroneals must be maintained with either dual reattachment or release. Control of the residual limb above the ankle is necessary, frequently incorporating an ankle foot orthosis (AFO) into a full-length shoe with filler. A spring-leaf dorsiflexion-assist AFO will allow for plantarflexion after heel strike, while providing assistance with dorsiflexion of the residual limb during swing phase.

Greene and Cary[30] have compared pediatric patients with ray, TMA, Chopart, Lisfranc, and midtarsal amputations with those with Syme amputation. The ray and TMA were superior to the Syme; the midfoot amputations that were properly balanced had better overall function, but needed greater adjustments for gait than the Syme group. Poorly balanced Chopart amputations were inferior to the Syme amputation.

Assumptions of how partial foot amputations and prostheses function have been called into question.[31] Such assumptions are based on static force analysis and GRFs seen in terminal stance in normal gait. CoP excursion data collected for Lisfranc and Chopart amputees do not support these assumptions, which places the GRF near where the metatarsal heads would have been during terminal stance. Clinically the peak GRF occurs well behind the terminal stump during terminal stance. It has been found that toe fillers, orthoses, and slipper sockets fitted to Lisfranc and transmetatarsal amputees were not able to restore effective foot length, due to a lack of a rigid couple between the residual limb and prosthesis as well as toe levers that are too flexible. Clamshell prostheses used for Chopart amputees, however, were found to effectively restore the effective foot length and a more normal peak GRF and gait pattern.[17]

SYME AMPUTATION

The Syme amputation disarticulates the ankle, and allows the amputee to bear weight directly on the residual limb.[29] Efficiency of gait is comparable to transtibial amputation (TTA) or TMA. It has been noted that Syme ankle disarticulations have a greater magnitude of propulsion and smaller metabolic cost of ambulation compared with midfoot amputees, although the midfoot amputees walk faster.[14] The GRF of a TMA differs entirely from the Syme. The shortened length of the residual foot serves as a smaller lever arm at push-off. Syme amputees have a decrease in speed of ambulation at 68% of able-bodied individuals, and 13% increased energy expenditure.

TRANSTIBIAL AMPUTATION

TTA is performed when more distal resections are not viable options, either because of bone or soft tissue compromise or poor distal circulation. Energy expenditure has been estimated to increase 9% to 30%[12–15] with TTA. Reduced cadence and shorter stride length has also been observed.[5] The length of the residual limb does not affect O_2 consumption or walking speed.[10,12] Restriction of ankle-joint mobility and loss of power caused by a lack of ankle plantarflexors can be substituted by recruitment of the hip and knee musculature.

Foot type does not tend to affect walking speed and energy cost with transtibial amputees[7-9]; however, socket type, specifically the contoured adducted trochanteric-controlled alignment method socket, has been shown to reduce oxygen consumption by 20% and increase walking speed by 10% compared with a traditional quadrilateral-shaped socket.[6] There is an increased risk of ulceration on the contralateral foot because of increased peak plantar pressures.[32] Mean peak plantar pressures have been noted to increase on the heel, with a higher-pressure time integral over the heel and the MTP regions.

SUMMARY

Amputations about the foot and ankle affect gait and energy consumption. More gait disturbances tend to be seen as amputation level becomes more proximal; however, loss of the MTP joints has a profound effect, regardless of the proximal level of amputation. Soft tissue balance is key to maximizing gait, particularly prevention of equinus and equinovarus deformity from unopposed plantarflexors. Orthotic, prosthetic, and shoe modifications can help minimize gait abnormalities; however, GRF and CoP alterations may still remain.

REFERENCES

1. Ziegler-Graham K, MacKenzie EJ, Ephraim PL, et al. Estimating the prevalence of limb loss in the United States: 2005 to 2050. Arch Phys Med Rehabil 2008;89: 422–9.
2. Moss SE, Klein R, Klein BE. The 14-year incidence of lower-extremity amputations in a diabetic population. The Wisconsin Epidemiologic Study of Diabetic Retinopathy. Diabetes Care 1999;22:951–9.
3. Dillingham TR, Pezzin LE, Shore AD. Reamputation, mortality, and health care costs among persons with dysvascular lower-limb amputations. Arch Phys Med Rehabil 2005;86:480–6.
4. Saunders JB, Inman VT, Eberhart HD. The major determinants in normal and pathological gait. J Bone Joint Surg Am 1953;35:543–58.
5. Kanade RV, van Deursen RW, Harding K, et al. Walking performance in people with diabetic neuropathy: benefits and threats. Diabetologia 2006;49:1747–54.
6. Gailey RS, Lawrence D, Burditt C, et al. The CAT-CAM socket and quadrilateral socket: a comparison of energy cost during ambulation. Prosthet Orthot Int 1993;17:95–100.
7. Casillas JM, Dulieu V, Cohen M, et al. Bioenergetic comparison of a new energy-storing foot and SACH foot in traumatic below-knee vascular amputations. Arch Phys Med Rehabil 1995;76:39–44.
8. Torburn L, Perry J, Ayyappa E, et al. Below-knee amputee gait with dynamic elastic response prosthetic feet: a pilot study. J Rehabil Res Dev 1990;27:369–84.
9. Torburn L, Powers CM, Guiterrez R, et al. Energy expenditure during ambulation in dysvascular and traumatic below-knee amputees: a comparison of five prosthetic feet. J Rehabil Res Dev 1995;32:111–9.
10. Gonzalez EG, Corcoran PJ, Reyes RL. Energy expenditure in below-knee amputees: correlation with stump length. Arch Phys Med Rehabil 1974;55:111–9.
11. Pinzur MS, Gold J, Schwartz D, et al. Energy demands for walking in dysvascular amputees as related to the level of amputation. Orthopedics 1992;15:1033–6 [discussion: 1036–7].

12. Waters RL, Perry J, Antonelli D, et al. Energy cost of walking of amputees: the influence of level of amputation. J Bone Joint Surg Am 1976;58:42–6.
13. Huang CT, Jackson JR, Moore NB, et al. Amputation: energy cost of ambulation. Arch Phys Med Rehabil 1979;60:18–24.
14. Pinzur MS, Wolf B, Havey RM. Walking pattern of midfoot and ankle disarticulation amputees. Foot Ankle Int 1997;18:635–8.
15. Molen NH. Energy-speed relation of below-knee amputees walking on a motor-driven treadmill. Int Z Angew Physiol 1973;31:173–85.
16. Pagliarulo MA, Waters R,·Hislop HJ. Energy cost of walking of below-knee amputees having no vascular disease. Phys Ther 1979;59:538–43.
17. Hirsch G, McBride ME, Murray DD, et al. Chopart prosthesis and semirigid foot orthosis in traumatic forefoot amputation. Comparative gait analysis. Am J Phys Med Rehabil 1996;75:283–91.
18. Catanzarti AR, Medicino RW, Haverstock B. Considerations for protection of the residual foot following transmetatarsal amputation. Wounds 1999;11: 13–20.
19. Lavery LA, Lavery DC, Quebedeax-Farnham TL. Increased foot pressures after great toe amputation in diabetes. Diabetes Care 1995;18:1460–2.
20. Dillon MP, Barker TM. Preservation of residual foot length in partial foot amputation: a biomechanical analysis. Foot Ankle Int 2006;27:110–6.
21. Mann RA, Poppen NK, O'Konski M. Amputation of the great toe. A clinical and biomechanical study. Clin Orthop Relat Res 1988;226:192–205.
22. Gianfortune P, Pulla RJ, Sage R. Ray resections in the insensitive or dysvascular foot: a critical review. J Foot Surg 1985;24:103–7.
23. Mueller MJ, Salsich GB, Bastian AJ. Differences in the gait characteristics of people with diabetes and transmetatarsal amputation compared with age-matched controls. Gait Posture 1998;7:200–6.
24. Mueller MJ, Allen BT, Sinacore DR. Incidence of skin breakdown and higher amputation after transmetatarsal amputation: implications for rehabilitation. Arch Phys Med Rehabil 1995;76:50–4.
25. Garbalosa JC, Cavanagh PR, Wu G, et al. Foot function in diabetic patients after partial amputation. Foot Ankle Int 1996;17:43–8.
26. Ayyappa E. Postsurgical management of partial foot and Syme's amputation. In: Lusardi M, editor. Orthotics and prosthetics in rehabilitation. Boston: Butterworth-Heinemann; 2000. p. 379–93.
27. Mueller MJ, Strube MJ, Allen BT. Therapeutic footwear can reduce plantar pressures in patients with diabetes and transmetatarsal amputation. Diabetes Care 1997;20:637–41.
28. Pinzur MS, Stuck RM, Sage R, et al. Syme ankle disarticulation in patients with diabetes. J Bone Joint Surg Am 2003;85:1667–72.
29. Lusardi MM, Nielsen CC. Foot and ankle prosthetics. In: Lusardi M, editor. Orthotics and prosthetics in rehabilitation. Boston: Butterworth-Heinemann; 2000. p. 386–93.
30. Greene WB, Cary JM. Partial foot amputations in children. A comparison of the several types with the Syme amputation. J Bone Joint Surg Am 1982;64: 438–43.
31. Dillon MP, Barker TM. Can partial foot prostheses effectively restore foot length? Prosthet Orthot Int 2006;30:17–23.
32. Kanade RV, van Deursen RW, Price P, et al. Risk of plantar ulceration in diabetic patients with single-leg amputation. Clin Biomech (Bristol, Avon) 2006;21: 306–13.

Shoes, Orthoses, and Prostheses for Partial Foot Amputation and Diabetic Foot Infection

Dennis J. Janisse, CPed[a,b,]*, Erick J. Janisse, CPed, CO[c]

KEYWORDS

• Shoes • Foot orthoses • Prostheses • Partial foot amputations

Amputations in patients with diabetes, while often preventable, are unfortunately a far too common outcome. Fifteen percent of diabetics will develop a foot ulcer over the course of their lifetime,[1] and foot ulcers are not to be taken lightly, as they are the precursor of 70% to 90% of all diabetic amputations.[2–7] Of special interest is the fact that partial foot amputations are nearly twice as common in the United States as either transtibial or transfemoral amputations.[8] The roles of the certified or licensed pedorthist, certified orthotist, and the certified prosthetist should not be undervalued in the prevention of diabetic foot complications (eg, amputations, revisions, and foot infections secondary to skin ulcerations) and in returning the patient a normal, active, and productive lifestyle in the event of an amputation. The primary goals of all three of these allied health professionals when working with partial foot amputees is to restore stability and function lost due to an amputation, facilitate energy-efficient gait, maintain support, and prevent any further complications.[9]

A certified pedorthist (a specialist trained in foot evaluation, shoe fitting and modification, and the fabrication and fitting of foot orthoses) can help prevent ulcerations and amputations by providing appropriate footwear and custom-made foot orthoses or prostheses. The pedorthist also employs modalities such as partial foot prostheses and shoe modifications to help protect the residual foot after an amputation in an effort to avoid reamputation.

[a] Department of Rehabilitation and Physical Medicine, Medical College of Wisconsin, Milwaukee, WI, USA
[b] National Pedorthic Services Incorporated, 7283 West Appleton Avenue, Milwaukee, WI 53216, USA
[c] National Pedorthic Services Incorporated, 660 North New Ballas Road, Saint Louis, MO 63141, USA
* Corresponding author. National Pedorthic Services Incorporated, 7283 West Appleton Avenue, Milwaukee, WI 53216.
E-mail address: djanisse@npsfoot.com

Foot Ankle Clin N Am 15 (2010) 509–523
doi:10.1016/j.fcl.2010.04.004
1083-7515/10/$ – see front matter. Published by Elsevier Inc.

Although there is little that shoes and foot orthoses can do to actually treat diabetic foot infections, they are invaluable tools in their prevention. Ill-fitting shoes are a prevalent cause of skin trauma that precedes the diabetic foot ulcers that can lead to partial foot amputation.[10] Areas of abnormally high plantar pressure and shear, two factors that can lead to diabetic skin ulcerations, are issues that may be addressed and alleviated with custom foot orthoses. Essentially, the key to avoiding diabetic foot infections is to prevent the opening of a portal of entry for infection to occur (eg, pressure ulcerations or minor traumatic skin wounds).

Through the use of lower limb orthoses or ankle foot orthoses (AFO) and prostheses, the orthotist helps restore functional gait to a person who has undergone a partial foot amputation surgery.[9,11] AFOs can be utilized to replace the lost lever arm of a transmetatarsal or hallux amputation.[9,11] They also can be used as offloading devices to decrease pressure on the plantar surface of the residual foot.

In regards to amputations in patients with diabetes, one often pictures the prosthetist fitting lower limb prostheses for transtibial amputations. The prosthetist also contributes significantly to the care of partial foot amputations, especially in the cases of a Chopart or Syme amputation. The prosthetist is also adept at fabricating aesthetically pleasing, realistic-looking partial foot prostheses for patients who are particularly concerned with the social implications or the stigma of a partial foot amputation, although, for reasons to be discussed later, some of these types of prostheses may be contraindicated for patients with diabetes or neuropathy.

With modern pedorthic, orthotic, and prosthetic techniques and devices, partial foot amputees can return to an as functional, or more functional, lifestyle than before the amputation.

PROPER SHOE SELECTION AND FIT

The importance of proper shoe selection and shoe fit cannot be underestimated. Therapeutic footwear plays an important role in the prevention of skin breakdown and subsequent infection, in preventing amputations, and in the care of the residual foot after partial foot amputation.[12–16]

Shoe selection in these cases necessarily needs to be based primarily on function, although fashion is important. It stands to reason that patients will be less likely to use the proper footgear if they strongly dislike its appearance.

In light of the fact that diabetic patients with a partial foot amputation also have a high incidence of ulceration, the functions of the shoe in the care of the foot after a partial foot amputation are as follows:

Protect the residual foot
Maintain foot position inside the shoe and reduce shear
Contribute to restoring normal gait
Accommodate an appliance such as a partial foot prosthesis, foot orthosis, or AFO.[15]

The shoe should be easily modifiable, as in many instances the prescription will call for external changes to the sole of the shoe. With advances in materials and adhesives, most athletic and comfort shoes are easily modified. It is quite simple for a technician to work with soles made of ethylene vinyl acetate (EVA), neoprene, or injection-molded polyurethane. Leather-soled shoes, while not difficult to modify, can become heavy and cumbersome when modified by adding lifts, shanks, or rocker soles. Rubber-soled shoes are not easily modified, nor are shoes with extraordinary so-called shock-absorbing features such as air bladders, pockets of gel, or springs.

Regardless of whether the patient has had an amputation, if someone has been diagnosed with sensory neuropathy, the upper portion of their shoe should be made of a material that is moldable, stretchable and breathable, such as like leather.[15] The interior lining of the shoe is important also. A lining of Plastazote or supple leather is desirable. Today, shoes are available commercially that are lined with materials that wick moisture away from the skin, such as Gortex, or have antibacterial properties, like X-static. These also warrant consideration for patients with diabetes.

High top shoes tend to work well for patients with transmetatarsal, Lisfranc and Chopart amputations, as they allow more interface with the foot and ankle, allowing the shoe to gain better purchase on the foot and leg.[11]

A shoe with a blucher opening allows for increased ease of donning and doffing and more adjustability over one with a balmoral opening. This type of opening allows for adjustability and space across the instep and forefoot areas, areas that can increase in volume after an amputation. A lace-to-toe, or surgical, opening works very well for patients with a partial foot amputation, although cosmetically it is typically not as well accepted as a blucher (**Fig. 1**).

Slip-on shoes loafers or dress shoes should be avoided, as most are, by their very nature, tight and restricting. Tight shoes should not be worn by patients with sensory neuropathy as they pose significant risk for increased surface pressure and shear on the foot; and the slip-on loafer or pump style shoe does not cover enough of the dorsum of the foot to make it practical for wear by a patient who has had transmetatarsal, Lisfranc or Chopart amputation. Shoes for patients with a partial foot amputation require some sort of closure system to be held on to the foot—laces, strap and buckle, or Velcro.

An in-depth shoe—that is, one that with additional room throughout the shoe and has one or more removable insoles[17]—is preferable when an orthopedic appliance such as an AFO, prosthesis, or foot orthosis will be worn.

Shoes are available in myriad styles, sizes, widths, and shapes. Finding a shoe that is perfectly matched to the patient, his or her feet, and his or her needs often requires the specialized skill set of a certified pedorthist. There is very little consistency in shoe sizing among manufacturers, making it almost impossible for the consumer to select a properly fitting shoe without guidance.

Some shoe styles are available in true widths, while others are not. If a shoe is manufactured in true widths, the base of the shoe is proportionally wider as the widths increase. This is not the case, however, with many commercial shoes, nor is it publicized by those manufacturers that do not offer true widths. Quite the opposite, in fact,

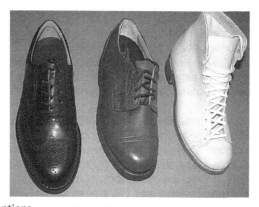

Fig. 1. Foot gear options.

is true, as many manufacturers label their shoes as being regular or wide width when they are not true widths at all. Only a shoe fitter with an intimate knowledge of his or her inventory can help guide a patient to an appropriate shoe.

A foot that has had a partial amputation can be challenging to fit properly. Shoes are designed so that in a normal foot the widest part of the foot, the ball, rests in the widest part of the shoe. In many cases, a partial foot amputation changes which area of the foot is the widest, or shortens it. This may require mismating of the shoes with a wider, shorter shoe on the affected side.

The topic of utilization of a custom-made short shoe versus use of a full-length shoe for the partial foot amputee has been debated over the years. Some authors have recommended the short shoe to provide a better fit for the residual foot.[18] The foreshortened shoe can be functional, effective, and comfortable, but it is often deemed unacceptable for cosmetic reasons.[9] Mueller and Strube[13] (1997) recommend the full-length shoe with a rigid rocker sole, as it was found to be more functional for a partial foot amputee after extensive testing of both types.[14]

SHEAR AND PLANTAR PRESSURE

Excessive shear and high peak plantar pressures long have been implicated as causal agents in the formation of plantar foot ulcers in persons with diabetic neuropathy. Luckily, therapeutic footwear decreases weight-bearing pressure and shear forces applied to the skin of the foot.[19] The plantar pressure gradient is another factor to consider.[20]

While much attention has been given to areas of high peak pressures as a predictor of foot ulcers, research has revealed that there is not a particularly high correlation between the two.[21–24] Reducing elevated pressure levels is important, but the need to reduce the duration of maximum pressure and shear stresses must not be overlooked.[25]

Diabetic ulcers frequently occur at locations where one has developed callusing.[26] The callusing is caused not solely from peak pressures, but from frictional shear forces.[27,28] It also has been documented that tissue breakdown occurs more rapidly when shear is increased.[29]

When walking, shear stresses act twice as frequently as pressure characteristically.[30] Because plantar shear is known to be a factor in the formation of preulcerative calluses, it must be taken into consideration when discussing diabetic foot ulcers. In also has been suggested that excessive shear may serve to damage the underlying tissues.[30] The damage done by repetitive friction load damage does not begin at the outermost layer of the skin; rather the friction causes shear forces between the layers of skin.[31]

In fact, it has been shown that diabetics with neuropathy experience increased plantar shear over a nondiabetic with no foot problems.[30]

Naylor demonstrated in the early 1950s that a peak perpendicular load by itself is not necessarily harmful. He established that the magnitude of repeated high peak pressures is worrisome because of how they enable and relate to peak friction loads.[32,33]

Perhaps the easiest way to reduce shear inside of a shoe is to be sure that the shoe size and shape are appropriate for the foot. If the shoe fits and is secured snugly on the foot via a tie or Velcro closure system, the foot does not shift inside the shoe as much. Proper fit is crucial, as a loose shoe and a tight shoe both have the potential to increase shear, friction, or pressure on the foot.

Another way to decrease friction and shear is to lubricate the surfaces moving against one another. This can be accomplished with the use of shear-reducing socks made from an acrylic blend fabric or other fiber that has a low coefficient of friction (COF). Traditional cotton socks have a relatively high COF, especially when damp. Keeping the feet and sock dry reduces shear, as do double socks. Double socks allow the shear to take place between the layers of socks as opposed to between the skin and sock or sock and insole.[34]

This lubrication also can be done using a special shear-reducing material on the interior of the shoe or on the surface of a foot orthosis or AFO under areas of high pressure or friction. A Teflon material called Shear Ban (Tamarack Habilitation Technologies Inc, MN, USA) is widely available to the orthotic, prosthetic, and pedorthic industry. The self-adhesive material can be adhered virtually anywhere inside of a shoe, brace, or prosthetic socket. It is also heat moldable.

When discussing reduction of peak plantar pressures, special attention often is given to the forefoot, as diabetic ulcers occur most frequently in this area.[20,21] It is for that reason that so much research has been devoted to reduction of forefoot pressures using shoes, rocker soles, and various types of foot orthoses.[35–39]

The peak pressure gradient, that is the spatial change in plantar pressure around the location of peak plantar pressure, is another pressure variable that warrants consideration. It has not been researched as extensively as peak plantar pressure, but Mueller and colleagues suggest that it may be a strong indicator of pending skin breakdown. Their research showed that the peak pressure gradient was significantly higher in the forefoot than in the heel even when compared with the peak plantar pressure.[20]

SHOE MODIFICATIONS

Rocker soles are probably the most commonly performed shoe modification.[15] They are especially useful when treating partial foot amputations and preventing and treating diabetic foot ulcerations and infections.

As the name suggests, a rocker sole serves to rock the foot from heel strike to toe-off without bending the foot or shoe. Essentially, the sole of the shoe is modified to resemble the base of a rocking chair or child's rocking horse. Generally speaking, the biomechanical effects of rocker soles are the restoration of lost motion in the foot and ankle due to pain, deformity, stiffness, or fusion, resulting in an overall improvement in gait and—of special significance to the diabetic foot—offloading plantar pressure on some part of the foot.[36] The rocker sole is considered to be the most effective way to offload the forefoot.[40] The rocker sole is also a logical method by which the center of pressure (CoP) can be progressed anteriorly past the distal end of the residual foot in a partial foot amputee.[41,42]

While there are several types of rocker soles, selection of the actual shape and type of rocker is based on the foot's individual needs.

It is necessary that two key terms be understood in order to discuss rocker soles: (1) the midstance, or the section of the rocker sole that is in contact with the ground when standing erect; and (2) the apex, or high point, of the rocker sole located at the distal end of the midstance.[43] These terms are illustrated in **Fig. 2**. Proper placement of the apex is the key to the success of the modification. The apex should be placed just proximal to the area in which pressure relief is needed. For example, if the desire is to offload the forefoot, the apex should be placed directly behind the metatarsal heads.

Many off-the-shelf walking shoes and running shoes are built with a mild rocker sole. This simple, generic rocker is often adequate for a foot that is not at risk. In fact, running shoes have been shown to be quite effective at reducing plantar pressures in the forefoot.[44] They provide some metatarsal head relief and gait assistance; however, for the patient who requires more relief or has deformity or neuropathy

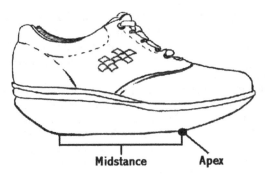

Midstance   **Apex**

Fig. 2. Rocker sole anatomy.

a custom rocker sole is indicated. An explanation of the six types of rocker soles follows[17,43]:

Mild rocker sole. This is the most widely used rocker sole. Utilizing a mild rock at the heel and at the toe, it relieves mild metatarsal head pressure and assists in gait by increasing forward propulsion. The other types of rocker soles are essentially variations on this most basic rocker (**Fig. 3**).

Heel-to-toe rocker sole. This rocker sole type is shaped with a more accentuated rocker angle at both the heel and toe. It is intended to dramatically increase propulsion at toe-off and decrease pressure on heel strike. It also reduces the need for ankle motion. This modification may be indicated for patients who have had

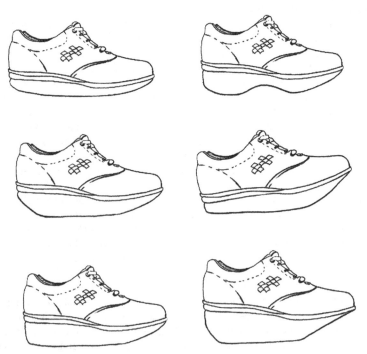

Fig. 3. Rocker sole types.

an ankle fusion or midfoot-level amputation, or use a solid ankle AFO (see **Fig. 3**).

Toe-only rocker sole. The toe-only rocker has no heel rock, only a rocker angle at the front with the midstance extending all the way to the back of the heel. This rocker is designed to increase weight bearing proximal to the metatarsal heads, provide a stable midstance, and reduce the need for toe dorsiflexion. It is useful for addressing forefoot issues in a patient who experiences difficulties with stability or proprioception (see **Fig. 3**).

Severe angle rocker sole. This rocker sole has a much more severe angle at the toe than the toe-only rocker sole. It has no heel rocker angle. This rocker sole significantly reduces weight-bearing pressures distal to the ball of the foot and is therefore indicated for extreme relief of metatarsal head or toe-tip ulcerations (see **Fig. 3**).

Negative heel rocker sole. The negative heel rocker is shaped with a rocker angle at the toe, with the heel height actually lower than the height of the sole under the ball of the foot. The purpose of this rocker sole is to relieve forefoot pressure by shifting it to the midfoot and heel. Because the effect is achieved in part by lowering the heel height, the height of the sole can be minimized, whereas other the other types of rockers may require the addition of material to the factory sole. The negative heel rocker is contraindicated for persons with balance or proprioception deficiencies or the inability to attain the necessary ankle dorsiflexion due to arthritis, fusion, or tendoachilles contracture (see **Fig. 3**).

Double rocker sole. This type of rocker sole technically consists of two shorter rocker soles with two short midstances. It is used to treat midfoot pathology. While unmodified shoes and shoes with the other types rocker soles actually increase pressure under the midfoot (when compared with barefoot), the double rocker sole does not.[35] This modification can be used to offload midfoot prominences such as a prominent fifth metatarsal base or those associated with a Charcot foot deformity (see **Fig. 3**).

The addition of an extended spring steel or carbon graphite composite shank is necessary in the partial foot amputee (**Fig. 4**). The 1 inch flat spring steel shank runs from the heel to the toe and is made of 16G or 18G steel.[9] This modification is performed in order to replace the toe-off lever arm that is lost due to a hallux or midfoot-level amputation and to prevent the shoe from deforming at the toe break and causing tissue damage to the residual foot.[9] The shank is inserted between the layers of the sole, extending from the heel to the toe of the shoe. The carbon composite shank is lighter in weight than the steel shank, but it susceptible to breakage when subjected to extreme repetitive forces, such as those found in the sole of a shoe to which a dorsiflexion-stop brace has been attached and is being used by a very large person.

It is commonly used in conjunction with a rocker sole and in fact can make the rocker sole more effective. The shank keeps the shoe from bending, thus reducing forces through the midfoot and forefoot. It strengthens the entire sole and shoe and maintains the continuity of the rocker sole.[43]

FOOT ORTHOSES

Custom-molded foot orthoses have been shown to reduce peak plantar pressures in the foot.[37,38,45] For a patient with sensory neuropathy, regardless of current amputation or infection status, the foot orthoses needs to be custom made. The primary

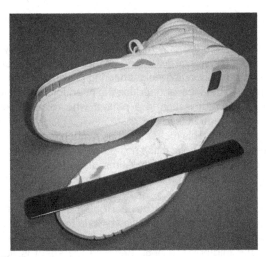

Fig. 4. Extended shank.

function of the device is pressure distribution via total contact between the foot orthoses and the foot or residuum. The goal is to eliminate or decrease areas of high peak pressure, high pressure sites that have an increased potential to develop skin breakdown.

This redistribution, and ideally equalization, of weight-bearing pressures over the plantar surface of the foot is achieved via the use of a total contact foot orthosis. This type of orthosis is constructed using a soft, conformable, cushioned top layer in conjunction with a firmer, supportive, but still forgiving, base layer. The materials are heated and formed over a positive model of the patient's foot. The contours of the plantar surface of the foot essentially are filled with material and then planed flat on the bottom, so that, in theory, when the patient stands on the orthosis the entire plantar surface of the foot is assuming weight-bearing responsibility.

One of the most commonly used top layer materials for patients with sensory neuropathy is Plastazote (Zotefoams plc, Surrey, England, UK). Plastazote, a moldable, static dissipative material, is a nitrogen-charged, closed-cell, cross-linked polyethylene foam. Its widespread use includes applications in the areas of shipping, athletic protective padding, building, military, and automotive industries. Its inert property, however, has made it particularly appealing to the medical industry over the years.

Used alone, Plastazote does not have a sufficiently long functional lifespan in a foot orthosis. When backed with a thin layer of polyurethane foam or EVA, it tends to endure longer under the repetitive stresses of walking. So common is the use of the aforementioned material combinations for foot orthosis fabrication in the pedorthic and orthotic industry, that several manufacturers offer prelaminated sheet stocks of them.

The base layer of a total contact foot orthosis needs to be one that will be supportive enough to adequately equalize plantar pressures but, because it is being made for an insensate foot, is still shock absorbing and, perhaps most importantly, easily adjustable. For this reason, the authors do not recommend a rigid thermoplastic or carbon composite base in a foot orthosis when being used in the treatment of a patient with diabetes or peripheral sensory neuropathy.

Potential base layer materials for semirigid total contact foot orthoses include EVA or cork with a Shore A durometer of approximately 50 to 60. The cork used in the construction of a foot orthosis of this type is not simply cork like that used in a wine bottle stopper. Depending on the manufacturer and physical properties desired by the practitioner, it is a combination of cork and any of the following: EVA, thermoplastic, latex rubber, and fiberglass. The cork composites, like EVA and Plastazote, are heat moldable. Although they are stiff at room temperature, they become quite pliable when heated and are easily molded to the model of the patient's foot.

Most cork composites and EVA also can be milled into the proper shape based on a computer scan of the foot when using a computer-aided design and computer-aided manufacturing (CAD-CAM) system. The firm base then is covered with a layer of softer EVA or Plastazote.

If not using a CAD-CAM system, the patient's foot is physically molded by the practitioner. Many techniques and materials can be used for obtaining the mold. Plaster, fiberglass, and wax can be wrapped around or molded directly to the patient's foot to capture the shape of the foot. Nowadays, it is common for a practitioner to use a block of closed-cell impression foam to capture the three-dimensional shape of the foot. The impression foam is lightweight and compresses easily. This method is quick and clean and produces an accurate negative mold of the foot.

The foam block is best utilized to obtain a semiweight-bearing mold of the foot, as this contour provides the greatest reduction of peak plantar pressures when compared with nonweight-bearing and full weight-bearing molds.[38] This method involves the practitioner seating the patient and aligning the hip, ankle, and knee at 90° angles. The practitioner manipulates the foot into a subtalar joint neutral or other desired position and then slowly and evenly depresses the foot into the foam. The patient is asked not to assist in the depressing of the foot (**Fig. 5**).

The negative mold (foam, plaster, fiberglass, or wax) then is filled with plaster, and the resultant positive model is used to fabricate the orthosis. The materials are heated in an oven and then vacuum-formed over the form of the foot. Once formed and cooled, a technician finishes the orthosis so that it may be placed into a shoe.

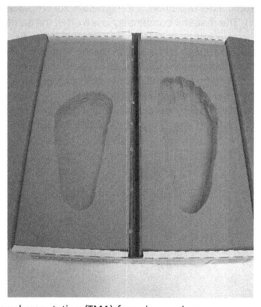

Fig. 5. Transmetatarsal amputation (TMA) foam impression.

The total contact orthosis at this stage should provide at least marginal plantar pressure redistribution and therefore some reduction of pressure under previously high pressure points. If more offloading is desired, the practitioner can add extrinsic posting to further reduce pressure in certain spots such as one or more metatarsal heads or a bony prominence such as the base of the fifth metatarsal. There are many preformed and shaped metatarsal pads that may be placed just proximal to the metatarsal heads to reduce pressure on them, or the pedorthist or orthotist may choose to make a custom metatarsal pad or metatarsal bar to be added to the orthosis.[39]

PARTIAL FOOT PROSTHESES

The main objective in amputation surgery for the surgeon is to salvage as much functional limb that will heal as possible, while the goal for the team of the surgeon, pedorthist, and prosthetist is to preserve and restore the patient's functional level.[9,11] The primary purpose of a partial foot prosthesis in a patient with diabetes is to protect the residual foot, with a secondary aim of restoring normal function and gait.

In oversimplified terms, equal pressure distribution is especially important in the partial foot patient, as peak plantar pressures rise exponentially as the amount of weight bearing surface area decreases, and more often than not, it is an insensate surface area to begin with. The issue of whether these tissues can handle the increased stress is why partial foot prostheses often are used in conjunction with an AFO—especially with a midfoot level amputation—to transfer the stresses to more proximal normal tissue.[46]

Like the foot orthoses discussed in the previous section, the partial foot prosthesis is used primarily to help evenly redistribute plantar pressures in the foot, reduce areas of high peak pressure, and decrease shear. Essentially, this is accomplished by fabricating a foot orthosis—in much the same manner as described previously—and adding an area of padding just distal to the end of the residual foot and then finishing it with a semirigid foam filler to maintain the foot's and the device's position within the shoe. The fabrication process is much the same whether the prosthesis is being fabricated for a hallux amputation, a ray resection, a transmetatarsal amputation, or a Lisfranc or Chopart amputation. The material combinations are often the same or similar to those used to fabricate the foot orthoses discussed previously (**Fig. 6**).

The loss of the hallux requires some sort of device to replace the lost lever arm for toe-off propulsion. This can be done via the use of an extended shank in the sole of the shoe, or it can be achieved by attaching a full-length carbon fiber footplate to, or incorporating it into, the partial foot prosthesis (**Fig. 7**).

Much has been written about the use of silicone or acrylic resin partial foot prosthesis (especially for Lisfranc and Chopart amputations) such as a Chicago boot or

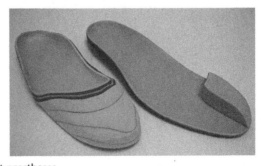

Fig. 6. Partial foot prostheses.

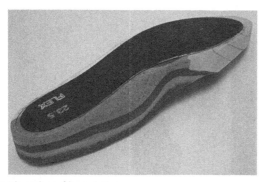

Fig. 7. TMA filler with carbon fiber plate.

a Lange prosthesis that slips over the residual foot, much like a sock or a shoe would.[9,11,46–49] These types of devices provide good cushion, stability, and excellent reduction in shear forces. Although they can be difficult to don and doff, they are cosmetically pleasing, and some may even be worn sans shoe. Because the focus of this article is on the diabetic foot, however, the authors recommend discretion when using these devices in the diabetic population, as these devices tend to be hot, which could make the foot perspire. They additionally do not permit any air circulation around the foot and may allow increased bacteria.[9]

The prosthesis for a Syme amputation is quite similar to that of the transtibial prosthesis except that the socket also serves as the shank. Because of the narrow space between the end of the residual limb and the floor, a standard prosthetic foot cannot be used without modification, as it would cause a leg length discrepancy. Therefore a Syme or Chopart-style prosthetic foot is used. Despite the fact that the end of the residual limb in this case can withstand more of the load than in the case of the transtibial amputation, it is still necessary to incorporate hydrostatic, or axial, offloading via patella tendon-bearing (PTB) features built into the device.

ANKLE FOOT ORTHOSES

Although there are many variations, the two basic AFO designs used for partial foot amputees are the solid ankle design, which allows no dorsiflexion or plantarflexion at the ankle, or a dorsiflexion-stop design, which allows full plantar flexion but no dorsiflexion past 90°.

One of the primary goals of AFO use is to progress the CoP past the distal end of the residual foot. To accomplish this, the AFO needs to incorporate three elements: a rigid lever arm to replace the lost toe lever, some method to control and halt forward progression of the tibia, and finally, a substantial socket capable of managing external torques resulting from increased forefoot loading.[50–52] Foot orthoses and partial foot prostheses do not allow the CoP to progress past the end of the residual foot until after the contralateral heel has made contact with the floor.[51,52] By contrast, several styles of AFOs do seem to normalize CoP excursion.[49,53]

An AFO also is used to restore medial–lateral stability that is lost due to a partial foot amputation.

Typically, the AFO will have a partial foot prosthesis built into the footplate of the brace. It also will be used in conjunction with a rocker sole (**Fig. 8**).

Solid ankle designs include a molded thermoplastic ankle foot orthosis, or MAFO. This device is easy to modify for a patient's changing needs.[11] This design provides

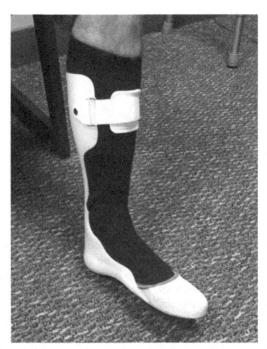

Fig. 8. AFO with filler.

good dorsiflexion and plantarflexion control as well as medial–lateral control. The advantage to the MAFO design is that it can be transferred easily from shoe to shoe by the patient (provided it is an appropriate shoe).

One way or another, the long toe-off lever arm should be incorporated. This can be accomplished either by extending the plantar footplate of the MAFO to the end of the shoe or by placing an extended shank in the sole of the shoe.

The addition of a PTB section to the MAFO can increase axial offloading on the residual foot. This weight reduction may be necessary to allow healing of or prevent ulcerations on the distal plantar aspect of the residual foot. The PTB modification provides for ambulation on a plantigrade foot without a high concentration of pressure on the distal end of the residual foot.[11] The PTB MAFO is probably the bulkiest and most confining of all AFO designs used for partial foot amputees.

Traditional double-upright, calf-lacer metal bracing systems also can be used for partial foot amputations. The advantage to this type of AFO is that there is no direct contact between the brace and the neuropathic foot. The brace is attached to the shoe externally, while the foot is protected inside of the shoe by a custom-made partial foot prosthesis. This design also may be altered to provide axial offloading by replacing the traditional leather calf-lacer with a Gillette-style calf lacer. The Gillette-style calf lacer is made with a thin layer of thermoplastic that is molded over a cast of the patient's leg for a stronger socket and a more intimate fit.

The double-upright AFO also can be set up to act as a dorsiflexion stop AFO. Other designs of the dorsiflexion stop include the MAFO and a lightweight, carbon fiber AFO. The former either can be a rear-entry design with a tall, shin guard-like anterior section, or it can be a traditional posterior shell articulated MAFO with a long, padded anterior shell; the carbon fiber AFO is typically a rear-entry design. Any time one is using a dorsiflexion stop design, a long padded anterior shell is required to spread the loads

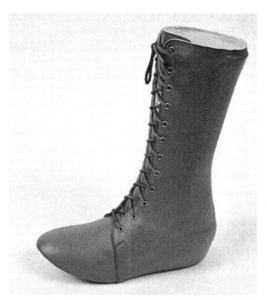

Fig. 9. Arizona AFO partial foot.

generated by rollover over as great a surface area as possible for the comfort and protection of the patient's skin over the tibia. The anterior shell also helps provide rotational control and stability.[11]

Another design that warrants consideration is a molded plastic and leather, total contact gauntlet design with an incorporated partial foot prosthesis, such as an Arizona AFO (Arizona AFO Inc, AZ, USA). Because of its total contact design, this type of AFO decreases pressure points on the skin (**Fig. 9**).

REFERENCES

1. Mancini L, Ruotolo V. The diabetic foot: epidemiology. Rays 1997;22(4):511–23.
2. Harvey D. New, improved Kerraboot: a tool for leg ulcer healing. Br J Community Nurs 2006;11(6):S26, S28–30.
3. Reiber GE, Vileikyte L, Boyko EJ, et al. Causal pathways for incident lower-extremity ulcers in patients with diabetes from two settings. Diabetes Care 1999;22:157–62.
4. Sedory Holzer SE, Camerota A, Martens L, et al. Costs and durations of care for lower-extremity ulcers in patients with diabetes. Clin Ther 1998;20:169–81.
5. Ollendorf DA, Kotsanos JG, Wishner WJ, et al. Potential economic benefits of lower-extremity amputation prevention strategies in diabetes. Diabetes Care 1998;21:1240–5.
6. Apelquist J, Bakker K, Van Houtum WH, et al. International consensus on the diabetic foot. Amsterdam (Netherlands): International Working Group on the Diabetic Foot; 1999.
7. Slater R, Ramot Y, Rapoport M. Diabetic foot ulcers: principles of assessment and treatment. Isr Med Assoc J 2001;3:59–62.
8. Owings M, Kozak L. Ambulatory and inpatient procedures in the United States, 1996. Vital Health Stat 13 1998;139:1–119.

9. Philbin TM, Leyes M, Sferra JJ, et al. Orthotic and prosthetic devices in partial foot amputations. Foot Ankle Clin 2001;6(2):215–28.

10. Reiber GE, Smith DG, Wallace C, et al. Clinical trial of footwear in patients with diabetes. JAMA 2002;287(19):2552–8.

11. Rheinstein J, Yanke J, Marzano R. Developing an effective prescription for a lower extremity prosthesis. Foot Ankle Clin North Am 1999;4(1):113–39.

12. Sanders LJ. Diabetes mellitus: prevention of amputation. J Am Podiatr Med Assoc 1994;84(9):483.

13. Mueller MJ, Strube MJ. Therapeutic footwear: enhanced function in people with diabetes and transmetatarsal amputation. Arch Phys Med Rehabil 1997;78: 952–6.

14. Mueller MJ, Strube MJ, Allen BT. Therapeutic footwear can reduce plantar pressures in patients with diabetes and transmetatarsal amputation. Diabetes Care 1997;20:637–41.

15. Janisse DJ, Janisse EJ. Pedorthic and orthotic management of the diabetic foot. Foot Ankle Clin 2006;11:717–34.

16. Mueller MJ. Therapeutic footwear helps protect the diabetic foot. J Am Podiatr Med Assoc 1997;87(8):360–4.

17. Janisse DJ. Prescription insoles and footwear. Clin Podiatr Med Surg 1995;1: 41–61.

18. Moore JW. Prostheses, orthoses, and shoes for partial foot amputees. Clin Podiatr Med Surg 1997;14:775–83.

19. Pinzur MS, Dart HC. Pedorthic management of the diabetic foot. Foot Ankle Clin 2001;6(2):205–14.

20. Mueller MJ, Zou D, Lott DJ. Pressure gradient as an indicator of plantar skin injury. Diabetes Care 2005;28(12):2908–12.

21. Yavuz M, Erdemir A, Botek G, et al. Peak plantar pressure and shear locations. Diabetes Care 2007;30(10):2643–5.

22. Armstrong DG, Peters EJ, Athanasiou KA, et al. Is there a critical level of plantar foot pressure to identify patients at risk for neurotrophic foot ulceration? J Foot Ankle Surg 1998;37:303–7.

23. Lavery LA, Armstrong DG, Wunderlich RP, et al. Predictive value of foot pressure assessment as part of a population-based diabetes disease management program. Diabetes Care 2003;26:1069–73.

24. Veves A, Murray HJ, Young MJ, et al. The risk of foot ulceration in diabetic patients with high foot pressure: a prospective study. Diabetologia 1992;35:660–3.

25. Dahmen R, Haspels R, Koomen B, et al. Therapeutic footwear for the neuropathic foot: an algorithm. Diabetes Care 2001;24(4):705–9.

26. Murray HJ, Young MJ, Hollis S, et al. The association between callus formation, high pressures and neuropathy in diabetic foot population. Diabet Med 1996; 13:979–82.

27. Goldblum RW, Piper WN. Artificial lichenation produced by a scratching machine. J Invest Dermatol 1954;22(5):405–15.

28. MacKenzie IC. The effects of frictional stimulation on mouse ear epidermis. J Invest Dermatol 1974;63(2):194–8.

29. Goldstein B, Sanders J. Skin response to repetitive mechanical stress: a new experimental model in pig. Arch Phys Med Rehabil 1998;79(3):265–72.

30. Yavuz M, Tajaddini A, Botek G, et al. Temporal characteristics of plantar shear distribution: relevance to diabetic patients. J Biomech 2008;41:556–9.

31. Sulzberger MB, Cortese TA, Fishman L, et al. Studies on blisters produced by friction. J Invest Dermatol 1966;47:456–65.

32. Naylor PFD. The skin surface and friction. Br J Dermatol 1955;67:239–48.
33. Naylor PFD. Experimental friction blisters. Br J Dermatol 1955;67:327–42.
34. Carlson JM. The friction factor. Orthokinetic Review 2001;1(7):1–3.
35. Janisse DJ, Brown D, Wertsch JJ, et al. Effects of rocker soles on plantar pressures and lower extremity biomechanics. Arch Phys Med Rehabil 2004;85:81–6.
36. Nawoczenski DA, Birke JA, Coleman WC. Effect of rocker sole design on plantar forefoot pressures. J Am Podiatr Med Assoc 1988;78:455–60.
37. Lavery LA, Vela SA, Fieischli JG, et al. Reducing plantar pressure in the neuropathic foot: a comparison of footwear. Diabetes Care 1997;20(11):1706–10.
38. Tsung BYS, Zhang M, Mak AFT, et al. Effectiveness of insoles on plantar pressure redistribution. J Rehabil Res Dev 2004;41(6A):767–74.
39. Hastings MK, Mueller MJ, Pilgram TK. Effect of metatarsal pad placement on plantar pressure in people with diabetes mellitus and peripheral neuropathy. Foot Ankle Int 2007;28(1):84–8.
40. Praet SF, Louwerens JK. The influence of shoe design on plantar pressures in neuropathic feet. Diabetes Care 2003;26:441–5.
41. Hansen AH. A biomechanist's perspective on partial foot prostheses. J Prosthet Orthot 2007;19(3S):80.
42. Janisse DJ. Pedorthic care of the diabetic foot. In: Bowker JH, Pfeifer MA, editors. Levin and O'Neal's the diabetic foot. 7th edition. St. Louis (MO): Mosby; 2008. p. 529–46.
43. Marzano R. Fabricating shoe modifications and foot orthoses. In: Janisse DJ, editor. Introduction to pedorthics. Columbia (MD): Pedorthic Footwear Association; 1998. p. 221–34.
44. Perry JE, Ulbrecht JS, Derr JA, et al. The use of running shoes to reduce plantar pressures in patients who have diabetes. J Bone Joint Surg 1995;77:1819–28.
45. Viswanathan V, Madhavan S, Gopalakrishna G, et al. Effectiveness of different types of footwear insoles for the diabetic neuropathic foot. Diabetes Care 2004; 27(2):474–7.
46. Condie DN, Stills ML. Partial-foot amputations: prosthetic and orthotic management. In: Bowker JH, Michael JW, editors. Atlas of limb prosthetics: surgical, prosthetic and rehabilitation principles. 2nd edition. Rosemont (IL): American Academy of Orthopaedic Surgeons; 1992. p. 403–12.
47. Lange LR. The lange silicone partial foot prosthesis. J Prosthet Orthot 1992; 4(1):56.
48. Burger H, Erzar D, Maver T, et al. Biomechanics of walking with silicone prosthesis after midtarsal (Chopart) disarticulation. Clin Biomech 2009;24(6):510–6.
49. Dillon MP, Barker TM. Comparison of gait of persons with partial foot amputation wearing prosthesis to matched control group: observational study. J Rehabil Res Dev 2008;45(9):1317–34.
50. Sessoms P, Fatone S, Hansen A. Case studies: gait analysis of persons with partial foot amputation walking barefoot and with dorsiflexion-stop ankle foot orthoses. Journal of Proceedings of the American Academy of Orthotists and Prosthetists Annual Meeting and Scientific Symposium 2009.
51. Dillon MP, Barker TM. Preservation of residual foot length in partial foot amputation: a biomechanical analysis. Foot Ankle Int 2006;27(2):110–6.
52. Dillon MP. Biomechanical models for the analysis of partial foot amputee gait [PhD thesis]. Queensland University of Technology Brisbane (Australia); 2001.
53. Dillon MP, Fatone S. Evidence note: the biomechanics of ambulation after partial foot amputation. Washington, DC: American Academy of Orthotists and Prosthetists; 2009.

Index

Note: Page numbers of article titles are in **boldface** type.

L

M

Moving?

Make sure your subscription moves with you!

To notify us of your new address, find your **Clinics Account Number** (located on your mailing label above your name), and contact customer service at:

Email: journalscustomerservice-usa@elsevier.com

800-654-2452 (subscribers in the U.S. & Canada)
314-447-8871 (subscribers outside of the U.S. & Canada)

Fax number: 314-447-8029

Elsevier Health Sciences Division
Subscription Customer Service
3251 Riverport Lane
Maryland Heights, MO 63043

*To ensure uninterrupted delivery of your subscription, please notify us at least 4 weeks in advance of move.